Understanding Fitness

Series Editor: Cara Acred

Volume 241

Independence Educational Publishers

First published by Independence Educational Publishers

The Studio, High Green

Great Shelford

Cambridge CB22 5EG

England

© Independence 2013

Photocopy licence

The material in this book is protected by copyright. However, the
purchaser is free to make multiple copies of particular articles for instructional
purposes for immediate use within the purchasing institution.
Making copies of the entire book is not permitted.

British Library Cataloguing in Publication Data

Understanding fitness. -- (Issues ; v. 241)

1. Health. 2. Obesity--Great Britain.

I. Series II. Acred, Cara.

306.4'613-dc23

ISBN-13: 9781 86168 639 8

Printed in Great Britain

MWL Print Group Ltd

Contents

Introduction

Understanding Fitness is Volume 241 in the **ISSUES** series. The aim of the series is to offer current, diverse information about important issues in our world, from a UK perspective.

ABOUT UNDERSTANDING FITNESS

Did you know 50% of people in the UK can't run 100 meters? With British people accused of being among the laziest in Europe, it is important to learn how we can embrace fitness, rather than shy away from it. Obesity is becoming a modern day epidemic, with many unaware of the dangers of being overweight or how to start tackling the problem. This book explores the concept of fitness and it's benefits, looks at the facts about obesity and looks at ways we can start to get active and be involved in fitness.

OUR SOURCES

Titles in the **ISSUES** series are designed to function as educational resource books, providing a balanced overview of a specific subject.

The information in our books is comprised of facts, articles and opinions from many different sources, including:

- Newspaper reports and opinion pieces

- Website fact sheets

- Magazine and journal articles

- Statistics and surveys

- Government reports

- Literature from special interest groups

A NOTE ON CRITICAL EVALUATION

Because the information reprinted here is from a number of different sources, readers should bear in mind the origin of the text and whether the source is likely to have a particular bias when presenting information (or when conducting their research). It is hoped that, as you read about the many aspects of the issues explored in this book, you will critically evaluate the information presented.

It is important that you decide whether you are being presented with facts or opinions. Does the writer give a biased or unbiased report? If an opinion is being expressed, do you agree with the writer? Is there potential bias to the 'facts' or statistics behind an article?

ASSIGNMENTS

In the back of this book, you will find a selection of assignments designed to help you engage with the articles you have been reading and to explore your own opinions. Some tasks will take longer than others and there is a mixture of design, writing and research based activities that you can complete alone or in a group.

FURTHER RESEARCH

At the end of each article we have listed its source and a website that you can visit if you would like to conduct your own research. Please remember to critically evaluate any sources that you consult and consider whether the information you are viewing is accurate and unbiased.

Physical activity and health

Facts and figures from Sustrans.

Definition

Physical activity includes all forms of activity, such as walking or cycling for everyday journeys, active play, work-related activity, active recreation such as working out in a gym, dancing, gardening or competitive sport.[1] Regular physical activity can reduce the risk of many chronic conditions including coronary heart disease, stroke, type 2 diabetes, cancer, obesity, mental health problems and musculoskeletal conditions.[1]

Targets

Everybody should aim to be active daily. For adults, the recommended amount is 150 minutes (2.5 hours) of moderate activity per week, in bouts of ten minutes or more. The overall amount of activity is more important than the type, intensity or frequency, and one way to achieve this is to do 30 minutes on at least five days a week.[1]

It is recommended that children over five should engage in at least 60 minutes (one hour) of moderate to vigorous intensity physical activity every day. Children under five who are capable of walking unaided should be physically active for at least 180 minutes (three hours), spread throughout the day.[1]

The Government has set a target in England and Wales for 70% of the population (in Wales, people up to the age of 65) to be 'reasonably active' by 2020 while in Scotland the target is for 50% of adults to achieve the minimum levels by 2022.[3,4,33]

According to the Welsh Assembly Government's Strategy for Physical Activity and Sport, *Climbing Higher,* physical activity 'can be broken down during the course of the day, because moderate physical activity, even if accumulated in short bouts, can achieve health-related benefit'.[3]

The four home countries' Chief Medical Officers have stated that the target, 150 minutes per week of moderate intensity activity will only be achieved by helping people to build activity into their daily lives. The 2004 report on physical activity says, 'for most people, the easiest and most acceptable forms of physical activity are those that can be incorporated into everyday life. Examples include walking or cycling instead of driving'.[2]

The report also states that 'the benefits of physical activity can be gained from activities that can be incorporated into everyday life such as regular brisk walking, using stairs and cycling. Physical activity does not have to be vigorous to confer protection'.[2]

Current levels

Physical activity levels are low in the UK: only 40% of men and 28% of women meet the minimum recommendations for physical activity in adults.[7]

In Scotland, '72% of women and 59% of men are not active enough for health', making physical inactivity the most common risk factor for CHD, more than obesity and smoking.[4]

The average level of inactivity in Wales is amongst the highest in the UK.[6] Only 36% of men and 22% of women meet the recommended levels of activity.[18]

Physical activity levels decline rapidly with increasing age. In England only 17% of men and 13% of women aged 65-74 are physically active.[5]

Scale of the physical inactivity problem

Physical inactivity is one of the leading causes of death in developed countries, responsible for an estimated 22-23% of CHD, 16-17% of colon cancer, 15% of diabetes, 12-13% of strokes and 11% of breast cancer.[8]

The cost of physical inactivity in England – including direct costs of treatment for the major lifestyle-related diseases, and the indirect costs caused through sickness absence – has been estimated at £8.2 billion a year. This does not include the contribution of inactivity to obesity which itself has been estimated at £2.5 billion annually.[2]

2,447 people in Scotland die prematurely each year due to physical inactivity. This is made up of 2,162 deaths from CHD (42% of total CHD deaths), 168 deaths from stroke (25% of total stroke deaths), and 117 deaths from colon cancer (25% of total colon cancer deaths).[4]

In Wales, the indirect costs of inactivity in terms of lost output and sickness absence, in addition to the direct costs of health care for entirely avoidable illness, comes to at least £500 million per annum, equating to around £200 for each person in Wales – every year.[6]

'A 10% increase in physical activity combined with a better diet could, conservatively, prevent 300 premature deaths each year and save the health service in Wales more than £25 million annually, with wider economic benefits in excess of £100 million annually'.[3]

'Increasing activity levels will contribute to the prevention and management of over 20 conditions and diseases including CHD, diabetes, cancer, positive mental health and weight management'.[9]

Physically active people have a 20-30% reduced risk of premature death and up to 50% reduced risk of major chronic disease such as CHD, stroke and cancer.[2]

3% of all disease burden in developed countries is caused by physical inactivity, and over 20% of CHD and 10% of stroke in developed countries is due to physical inactivity.[8]

Regular moderate physical activity, including walking and cycling, can help prevent and reduce the risk of:

Cardiovascular disease (CVD)

⇨ In the UK around 36% of people die from CVD – the main forms are Coronary Heart Disease (CHD) (half of all CVD deaths) and stroke (around a quarter).[11]

⇨ CHD is the leading cause of death in the UK, causing 101,000 deaths a year. One in five men and one in six women die from the disease. Almost one million people living in the UK have had a heart attack.[11]

⇨ 'CVD, including heart disease and stroke, and cancer are the major causes of death in England, together accounting for almost 60% of premature deaths'.[9]

⇨ Death rates from CHD in the UK are highest in Scotland and the North of England and lowest in the South of England.[11]

⇨ An estimated 4.2% of males and 3.0% of females in Scotland have CHD.[15]

⇨ CVD is estimated to cost the UK economy just under £26 billion a year and CHD over £7.9 billion a year.[11]

⇨ Inactive and unfit people have almost double the risk of dying from CHD compared with more active and fit people.[2]

Cancer

⇨ 'People who are physically active tend to have a lower risk of cancer ... the higher the level of physical activity or fitness, the lower the overall risk of cancer. Moderate to vigorous intensity activity appears to be most beneficial. Frequency is also a factor: more frequent physical activity has been associated with greater risk reductions'.[2]

⇨ Cancer and CVD are responsible for around 60% of preventable deaths in England.[9]

⇨ 137 people per 100,000 die from cancer in deprived areas in England compared to the England average of 119 people per 100,000.[10]

⇨ It is estimated that 25% of all deaths from colon cancer in Scotland are attributable to physical inactivity.[16]

⇨ Physical activity is associated with a reduced risk of breast cancer in women after the menopause. Women with higher levels of physical activity have about a 30% lower risk of breast cancer than the least active.[16]

⇨ Inactive people have a 3.6% higher risk of colon cancer.[5]

⇨ Physical activity has a clear protective effect on colon cancer. The most active individuals have, on average, a 40-50% lower risk than the least active.[16]

⇨ 'Physical activity can have an indirect effect through its role in the prevention of obesity which, in the USA, has been estimated to result in 10% of all-cause cancer'.[2]

Physical activity (expenditure of calories, raised heart rate)		
Everyday activity:	**Active recreation:**	**Sport:**
Active travel (cycling/ walking)	Recreational walking	Sport walking
Heavy housework	Recreational cycling	Regular cycling
Gardening	Active play	Swimming
DIY	Dance	Exercise & fitness training
Occupational activity (active/manual work)		Structured competitive activity
		Informal sport
		Individual pursuits

Source: Start Active, Stay Active, *Department of Health, Physical Activity, Health Improvement and Protection, 11 July 2011 © Crown copyright 201[?]*

Obesity and overweight

⇨ Obesity 'doubles the risk of all-cause mortality, coronary heart disease, stroke and type 2 diabetes, and increases the risk of some cancers, musculoskeletal problems and loss of function, and carries negative psychological consequences'.[2]

⇨ 'Obesity reduces life expectancy on average by nine years'.[20]

⇨ In England, the proportion of adults categorised as obese (BMI over 30) increased from 13.2% of men in 1993 to 23.7% in 2006 and from 16.4% of women in 1993 to 24.2% in 2006. Around 44% of men and 35% of women in England are overweight.[7]

⇨ More than two-thirds of women and three-quarters of men aged 55-74 in England, are overweight or obese.[2]

⇨ The prevalence of obesity in two to ten-year-olds increased from 9.6% to 17.1% among boys, and from 10.3% to 13.2% among girls between 1995 and 2006.[7]

⇨ In Wales, 37% of adults are overweight and 18% of adults are obese.[18]

⇨ In Scotland around 22% of men and 24% of women are obese. 64% of men and 57% of women are overweight.[19]

⇨ Overweight and obesity are increasing rapidly. In England the percentage of adults aged 16-64 who are obese has doubled in the past decade.[11]

⇨ 'It is likely that for many people, 45–60 minutes of moderate-intensity physical activity a day is necessary to prevent obesity'.[9]

⇨ Rates of obesity are estimated to rise, by 2035, to 47% and 36% for adult men and women, respectively. By 2050, 60% males and 50% females could be obese.[30]

⇨ 'Physical activity that can be incorporated into everyday life – such as walking and cycling – appears to be as effective for weight loss as supervised exercise programmes'.[2]

⇨ The total annual cost to the NHS of overweight and obesity (i.e. the treatment of obesity and its consequences) is estimated at £2 billion, and the total impact on employment may be as much as £10 billion.[30]

⇨ By 2050, the NHS cost of overweight and obesity could rise to £9.7 billion, with the wider cost to society being £49.9 billion (at today's prices).[30]

Diabetes

Diabetes mellitus is a condition in which the amount of glucose (sugar) in the blood is too high because the body cannot use it properly. There are two types of diabetes, type 1 (insulin dependent) which accounts for 5% to 10% of the diagnoses and type 2 (non insulin dependent) which is much more prevalent and accounts for 90% to 95% of cases. type 2 is closely linked to obesity.

⇨ 'People with diabetes have a higher chance of developing certain serious health problems, including heart disease, stroke, high blood pressure, circulation problems, nerve damage, and damage to the kidneys and eyes. The risk is particularly high for people with diabetes who are also very overweight, who smoke or who are not physically active.' Regular physical activity helps reduce the risk of developing any of these complications.[21]

⇨ 5.6% of men and 4.2% of women in England have diagnosed diabetes – type 2 accounts for most cases.[7]

⇨ 3% of men and 0.7% of women are likely to have undiagnosed diabetes.[7]

⇨ In total there are likely to be 2.5 million adults in the UK with diabetes.[11]

⇨ 5% of adults in Wales reported being treated for diabetes.[18]

⇨ It is estimated that 161,000 people in Scotland are affected by type 2 diabetes (3.2% of the population).[16]

⇨ The prevalence of diagnosed diabetes has more than doubled in men, and increased by 85% in women since 1991.[11]

⇨ Prevalence of diabetes in England almost doubled between 1994 and 2003.[7]

⇨ The number of people with diabetes is set to almost double over the next 20 years.[22]

⇨ 'Physically active people have a 33-50% lower risk of developing type 2 diabetes compared to inactive people'.[2]

⇨ Regular physical activity can reduce the risk of developing type 2 diabetes by up to 64% in those at high risk of developing the disease.[23]

Stroke

Stroke is the term used to describe the effects of an interruption of the blood supply to a localised area of the brain. If part of the brain is deprived of blood, brain cells are damaged or die. This causes a number of different effects, depending on the part of the brain affected and the amount of damage to brain tissue.

⇨ Stroke is the third most common cause of death in England and Wales after heart disease and cancer and the leading cause of disability in the UK.[24]

⇨ Around 100,000 people in England and Wales have a first stroke each year – one every five minutes.[24]

⇨ At least 300,000 people are living with moderate to severe disabilities as a result of a stroke.[24]

⇨ It is estimated that 26% of all deaths from stroke in Scotland are attributable to physical inactivity.[16]

⇨ Stroke costs the UK economy £7 billion a year in health and social costs.[11]

⇨ In England the prevalence of stroke in women increased from 1.6% in 1994 to 2.2% in 2006; similarly, the overall rate of stroke in men has risen from 1.8% to 2.4%.[7]

⇨ 'The majority of studies report that those who do regular to light to moderate activity have a lower incidence of stroke compared with those who are inactive, and some data suggest that vigorous activity confers no additional benefit'.[2]

Further facts and figures are available from the Stroke Association.[24]

Mental health problems

⇨ 'One in four people will experience some kind of mental health problem in the course of a year'.[25]

⇨ 'One in four of us will experience a mental health problem at some point in our lives. Each year more than 250,000 people are admitted to psychiatric hospitals'.[26]

⇨ Regular physical activity improves mood, helps relieve depression, and increases feelings of well-being. A survey carried out by the charity Mind found that 83% of people with mental health problems looked to physical activity to help lift their mood.[27]

⇨ 'Physical activity is effective in the treatment of clinical depression and can be as successful as psychotherapy or medication, particularly in the longer term'.[2]

⇨ 'Physical activity can be considered for its therapeutic effects on mental illness, and also for its impact on mental health in the general population'.[2]

⇨ Physical activity can help reduce physiological reactions to stress, improve sleep, reduce anxiety.[1]

⇨ Rhythmic aerobic forms of exercise – including brisk walking and cycling, appear to be most consistently effective.[1]

⇨ 'Regular physical activity reduces the risk of depression and has positive benefits for mental health including reduced anxiety, and enhanced mood and self-esteem'.[9]

⇨ Physical activity may improve at least some aspects of cognitive function that are important for tasks of daily living, and is also associated with a reduced risk of developing problems of cognitive impairment in old age.[16]

High blood pressure

Blood pressure is the pressure of blood in your arteries. The higher your blood pressure the greater your risk of developing narrowed arteries which can lead to heart problems and strokes. Exercising helps lower blood pressure.

⇨ In England 33.5% of men and 28.8% of women have hypertension.[7]

⇨ 42% of women aged 55-64 in the UK have high blood pressure, and two thirds of women aged 65-74.[11]

⇨ Among adults in Wales, 16% of males and 20% of females reported being treated for high blood pressure with the greatest proportion being over 65 years of age.[18]

⇨ People with a history of high blood pressure have almost twice the risk of a heart attack compared to those with no history of high blood pressure.[11]

⇨ Participating in physical activity helps lower blood pressure.[28]

⇨ 'High blood pressure can be both prevented and treated by physical activity'.[2]

⇨ Regular physical activity prevents high blood pressure and reduces blood pressure in people with hypertension.[23]

Musculoskeletal health – osteoporosis and osteoarthritis

This is the loss of bony tissue, resulting in bones that are weak and brittle and liable to fracture. This occurs most commonly in old people, particularly

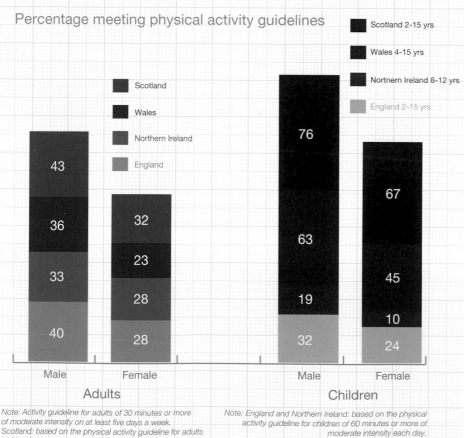

Percentage meeting physical activity guidelines

Scotland 2-15 yrs
Wales 4-15 yrs
Northern Ireland 8-12 yrs
England 2-15 yrs

Scotland
Wales
Northern Ireland
England

Adults — Male: 43, 36, 33, 40; Female: 32, 23, 28, 28
Children — Male: 76, 63, 19, 32; Female: 67, 45, 10, 24

Note: Activity guideline for adults of 30 minutes or more of moderate intensity on at least five days a week. Scotland: based on the physical activity guideline for adults of 30 minutes or more of moderate intensity on most days of the week.

Note: England and Northern Ireland: based on the physical activity guideline for children of 60 minutes or more of moderate intensity each day. Wales and Scotland: based on the physical activity guideline for children of 60 minutes or more of moderate intensity on five days a week.

Source: Start Active, Stay Active, Department of Health, Physical Activity, Health Improvement and Protection, 11 July 2011
© Crown copyright 2011

women, but it can also result from longer-term steroid therapy, infection or injury.

⇨ The health and social care costs of osteoporosis in the UK amount to £1.7-£1.8 billion a year.[16]

⇨ 'Physical activity can increase bone mineral density in adolescents, maintain it in young adults, and slow its decline in old age'.[2]

⇨ Physical activity can prevent up to 25% of falls by regulating the production and circulation of hormones, improving balance and developing muscle power.[2]

⇨ Moderate daily general physical activity, especially walking, may be associated with a lower risk of subsequent osteoarthritis, especially in women.[2]

⇨ Increasing activity levels has beneficial effects on musculoskeletal health, reducing the risk of osteoporosis, back pain and osteoarthritis.[8]

⇨ Physical activity can help prevent osteoporosis; daily physical activity, especially walking, may be associated with a lower risk of subsequent osteoarthritis, especially among women.[16]

⇨ Physical activity can help reduce the risk of falling, and therefore fractures, among older people.[16]

⇨ A broad range of physical activities can reduce pain, stiffness and disability, and increase general mobility, gait, function, aerobic fitness and muscle strength in older adults with osteoarthritis.[16]

⇨ The above information is reprinted with kind permission from Sustrans. Please visit www.sustrans.org.uk for further information.

© Sustrans 2012

References

1. Department of Health (2011). Start Active, Stay Active: A report on physical activity for health from the four home countries' Chief Medical Officers

2. Department of Health (2004). At least five a week – evidence on the impact of physical activity and its relationship to health – a report from the Chief Medical Officer

3. Welsh Assembly Government (2003). Climbing Higher – Sport and Active Recreation in Wales Strategy for Consultation

4. Physical Activity Task Force (2003). Let's Make Scotland More Active – A Strategy for Physical Activity, Scottish Executive

5. National Centre for Social Research et al (2004). Health Survey for England 2003

6. Welsh Assembly Government (2005). Climbing Higher – The Welsh Assembly Government Strategy for Sport and Physical Activity

7. NHS Information Centre (2008). Health Survey for England 2006. CVD and risk factors adults, obesity and risk factors children

8. World Health Organization (2002). The World Health Report 2002 – Reducing Risks, Promoting Healthy Life

9. Department of Health (2005). Choosing Activity: a physical activity action plan

10. Government National Sustainable Development Indicators 2006

11. British Heart Foundation (2007). Coronary Heart Disease Statistics

12. Scottish Executive (2005). Delivering for Health

13. Department of Health, HIU: Health Inequalities PSA Target

15. ISD Scotland CHD Statistics

16. Health Scotland (2007). Active for Later Life: Promoting physical activity with older people. A resource for agencies and organisations

17. Department of Health (2004). Health Survey for England 2004

18. Statistical Directorate National Assembly for Wales (2005). Welsh Health Survey 2004/05

19. Scottish Executive Statistics (2005). 2003 Scottish Health Survey

20. Department of Health (2005). Delivering Choosing Health: making healthier choices easier

21. Muslim Health Network

22. Diabetes UK (2004). Diabetes in the UK 2004

23. Sport England (2007). Active Design: Promoting opportunities for sport and physical activity through good design

24. Stroke Association

25. Mental Health Foundation

26. MIND

27. MIND 2001

28. Blood Pressure Association

29. Department of Health (2008). Healthy Weight, Healthy Lives, a Cross-Government Strategy for England

30. Government Office for Science (2007). Foresight: Tackling obesity – Future Choices

31. Welsh Assembly Government (2006). Welsh Health Survey 2005/06

32. Drakeford, M. (2006). Health Policy in Wales: Making a difference in conditions of difficulty, Critical Social Policy 26, 543–561

33. Strategy Unit (2002). Game Plan: a strategy for delivering Government's sport and physical activity objectives

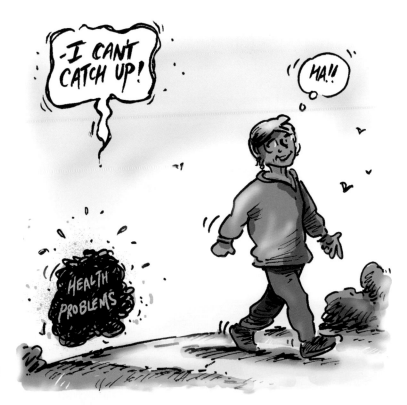

Start active, stay active

A report on physical activity for health from the four home countries' Chief Medical Officers.

These guidelines are issued by the four Chief Medical Officers (CMOs) of England, Scotland, Wales and Northern Ireland. They draw on global evidence for the health benefits people can achieve by taking regular physical activity throughout their lives. Even relatively small increases in physical activity are associated with some protection against chronic diseases and an improved quality of life.

Key features of this report include:

⇨ a life-course approach

⇨ a stronger recognition of the role of vigorous intensity activity

⇨ the flexibility to combine moderate and vigorous intensity activity

⇨ an emphasis upon daily activity

⇨ new guidelines on sedentary behaviour.

Each of us should aim to participate in an appropriate level of physical activity for our age.

Early years (under-fives)

Physical activity should be encouraged from birth, particularly through floor-based play and water-based activities in safe environments.

Children of pre-school age who are capable of walking unaided should be physically active daily for at least 180 minutes (three hours), spread throughout the day.

All under-fives should minimise the amount of time spent being sedentary (being restrained or sitting) for extended periods (except time spent sleeping).

Children and young people (five to 18 years)

All children and young people should engage in moderate to vigorous intensity physical activity for at least 60 minutes and up to several hours every day.

Vigorous intensity activities, including those that strengthen muscle and bone, should be incorporated at least three days a week.

All children and young people should minimise the amount of time spent being sedentary (sitting) for extended periods.

Adults (19–64 years)

Adults should aim to be active daily. Over a week, activity should add up to at least 150 minutes (two and a half hours) of moderate intensity activity in bouts of ten minutes or more – one way to approach this is to do 30 minutes on at least five days a week.

Alternatively, comparable benefits can be achieved through 75 minutes of vigorous intensity activity spread across the week or a combination of moderate and vigorous intensity activity.

Adults should also undertake physical activity to improve muscle strength on at least two days a week.

All adults should minimise the amount of time spent being sedentary (sitting) for extended periods.

Older adults (65+ years)

Older adults who participate in any amount of physical activity gain some health benefits, including maintenance of good physical and cognitive function. Some physical activity is better than none, and more physical activity provides greater health benefits.

Older adults should aim to be active daily. Over a week, activity should add up to at least 150 minutes (two and a half hours) of moderate intensity activity in bouts of ten minutes or more – one way to approach this is to do 30 minutes on at least five days a week.

For those who are already regularly active at moderate intensity, comparable benefits can be achieved through 75 minutes of vigorous intensity activity spread across the week or a combination of moderate and vigorous activity.

Older adults should also undertake physical activity to improve muscle strength on at least two days a week.

Older adults at risk of falls should incorporate physical activity to improve balance and co-ordination on at least two days a week.

All older adults should minimise the amount of time spent being sedentary (sitting) for extended periods.

Conclusion

This report sets out clearly what people need to do to benefit their health and can help them to understand the options for action that fit their own busy lives. There now needs to be careful and planned translation of these guidelines into appropriate messages for the public, which relate to different situations.

11 July 2011

⇨ The above information is reprinted from the *Start Active, Stay Active* report issued by the four Chief Medical Officers (CMOs) of England, Scotland, Wales and Northern Ireland. Please visit www.bhfactive.org.uk for further information.

British people among laziest in Europe

Britons are among the laziest people in Europe, according to a study which found that almost two thirds of adults are putting their health at risk through a lack of exercise.

By Nick Collins, science correspondent

Only Malta and Serbia saved British people the title of the most slothful in the continent by a new study into global levels of activity.

Some 63 per cent of adults in this country are failing to meet health guidelines which advocate at least 30 minutes of moderate exercise, such as brisk walking, five times a week or 20 minutes of more vigorous activity three times a week.

Falling below this target can raise the risk of conditions like heart disease, diabetes and certain types of cancer by 20 to 30 per cent, doctors warn.

Our lethargy is double the global average and the eighth worst of the 122 countries studied, which collectively account for 89 per cent of the world's population.

Malta was the laziest country worldwide, with 72 per cent of adults classified as physically inactive, but Britain (63%) far outstretched other countries like the USA (41%), France (33%) and Greece (16%).

One third of adults across the world and four in five teenagers are physically inactive according to the study, which was based on self-reported data.

Pedro Hallal of Universidade Federal de Pelotas in Brazil, who led the study, said: 'In most countries, inactivity rises with age and is higher in women than in men. Inactivity is also increased in high-income countries.'

The study is part of a wider series on physical activity published in the latest issue of the *Lancet* journal.

In a separate paper, researchers from Harvard Medical School reported that lack of exercise now ranks alongside smoking and obesity in its contribution to disease.

Physical inactivity was responsible for 5.3 million of the 57 million deaths worldwide in 2008 including six to ten per cent of cases of heart disease, type 2 diabetes, breast and colon cancer, they estimated.

Professor Mark Batt, President of the UK Faculty of Sport and Exercise Medicine, said: 'Physical activity is the most prevalent modifiable risk factor for chronic disease, and this is one of the many reasons we need to work harder to promote the advantages of exercise across the country.

'Physical activity should be ingrained in daily routines and our way of life, but this is simply not the case at the moment.'

18 July 2012

⇨ The above article originally appeared in *The Telegraph* and is reprinted with permission. Please visit www.telegraph. co.uk for further information.

New research shows that healthy teenagers are happy teenagers

Research into adolescent health behaviour by Dr Cara Brooks, Senior Research Officer at the Institute for Social and Economic Research at the University of Essex, used information from Understanding Society, a long-term study of 40,000 UK households funded by the Economic and Social Research Council (ESRC).

Dr Brooks looked at the responses of 5,000 young people aged ten to 15 to questions about their health-related behaviours and levels of happiness. The results show that:

⇨ Young people who never drank any alcohol were between four and six times more likely to have higher levels of happiness than those who reported any alcohol consumption.

⇨ Young people who smoked were about five times less likely to have high happiness scores compared to those who never smoked.

⇨ Higher consumption of fruit and vegetables and lower consumption of crisps, sweets and fizzy drinks were both associated with high happiness.

⇨ The more hours of sport young people participated in per week, the happier they were.

Researchers at the Institute for Social and Economic Research at the University of Essex believe the data shows that unhealthy behaviours such as smoking, drinking alcohol and taking no exercise are closely linked to substantially lower happiness scores among teenagers, even when factors such as gender, age, family income and parent's education are taken into account.

The researchers argue that 'there are clear long-term links between health-related behaviours and well-being in adulthood. Helping young people to reduce damaging health choices as they start making independent decisions is important in order to reduce the number of adults at risk from chronic disease because of their low well-being and poor health-related behaviours.'

The PSHE Association believes that this research is important for schools to understand and continues to press for PSHE education to be made a statutory entitlement for all children and young people in schools taught by properly trained, confident and competent teachers.

The findings above are taken from the article 'Happiness and health-related behaviours in adolescence' from the *Understanding Society: Findings 2012* report.

5 March 2012

⇨ The above information is reprinted with kind permission from the PSHE Association. Please visit www.pshe-association.org.uk for further information.

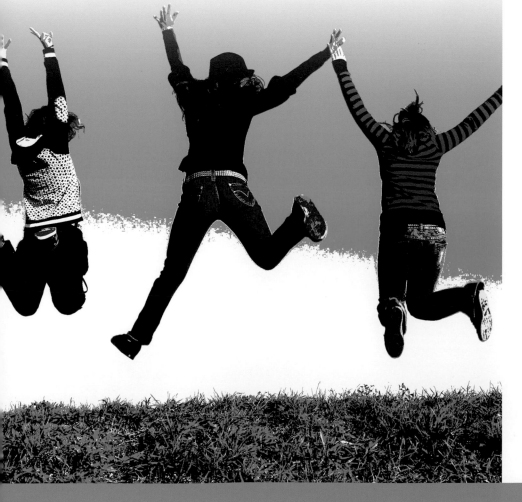

Fred Turok, chair of the Physical Activity Network talks about the Olympic legacy

Information from the Department of Health.

What an incredible two weeks of sport. The Games have had everything: passion, excitement, enthusiasm and more success than anyone could have imagined. All the world's top athletes competed in London and Team GB won over 50 medals, finishing an unbelievable 3rd in the medal rankings; an amazing achievement!

However, before we all get carried away with celebration and festivity, a small word of caution: in my opinion, for the Games to really be judged a national success, we must deliver on our promise to create a sustainable, long-term health legacy and encourage the nation to get more active, not just in the next few months but for years to come. This is not just important for us to successfully nurture another generation of gold medallists but critical for the country's health and well-being.

The Responsibility Deal Physical Activity Network will have an important role to play in this – by facilitating partnerships between businesses, the third sector and the public sector to harness the enthusiasm generated by the Games.

In all my years promoting physical activity, we have never had such a good opportunity to embrace sport and embed an active lifestyle into the DNA of the nation. Since the Games began, Olympic fever has spread into swimming pools, badminton courts and parks up and down the country. It's been incredible. Yet history suggests that creating a lasting legacy will require real focus: the evidence shows that no host has ever been able to achieve any kind of real legacy.

We can't let this happen. With an ageing population, concerns about the levels of physical activity within schools, and rising levels of obesity and type 2 diabetes the health consequences are literally too dire. A recent *Lancet* study found that physical inactivity now causes as many deaths across the world as smoking; accounting for one in ten deaths globally from diseases such as heart disease and cancer. It named Britain as the third most inactive country in Europe, with 63% of adults not meeting minimum levels of physical activity. It called the situation an inactivity 'pandemic' that is responsible for the death of millions of people every year that could have been prevented.

It is estimated that there are currently 2.9 million people with diabetes in the UK. By 2025 this will reach five million people; the equivalent of more than 400 people developing the disease every day, over 17 every hour and around three people every ten minutes. A total of 61.3% of adults are either overweight or obese and even more worryingly 33.3% of all ten to 11-year-olds. According to the Chief Medical Officer, physical activity can reduce the prevalence of chronic conditions such as type 2 diabetes, obesity and stroke by between 30-40%.

A societal problem needs to be tackled through a societal approach. This excludes nobody. We must all play our part. There is a role for both athletes and spectators; head teachers and parents; employees and employers; doctors and patients; students and seniors; central and local government. The cost of obesity is expected to reach an exorbitant £50 billion per year by 2050. If we want our children to have an NHS free at the point of use then we need to change our lifestyles and as a nation become more active.

The provision of physical activity in schools is currently in the spotlight, with figures showing that whilst 9.8% of our children enter primary school as obese, twice as many (18.7%) leave primary schools as obese. Initiatives that provide 'sport volunteers' to local schools must be rolled out nationwide. Exercise is by far the most cost-effective and beneficial medicine that exists. It has no side-effects and usually encourages healthier all-round behaviour. Over 835,000 people visit their local GP practice every day – our GPs have a vital role in encouraging their patients to incorporate activity into their daily lives. Physical activity programmes designed around one-on-one motivational support and counselling have proven successful – they must be commissioned more broadly. Through the Responsibility Deal there are some great examples of business supporting the promotion of physical activity, such as Asda delivering a series of summer events for families aimed at encouraging physical activity within deprived communities – these have to be expanded.

For these Olympic and Paralympic Games to be deemed a real success, we must deliver on our commitment to achieve a real health legacy. Our athletes may have inspired us to get out and exercise today, but we must remain active tomorrow and the day after. This goes beyond a two-week sporting showcase. It is a national crisis. One that I really hope we can overcome.

13 August 2012

⇨ The above information is reprinted with kind permission from the Department of Health. Please visit www.dh.gov.uk for further information.

London 2012 Olympic Games legacy 'non-existent', says medalist Liz McColgan

Olympic medalist Liz McColgan has said she fears that a generation of aspiring athletes will see no benefit from any 'legacy' from the London Games.

By Andy Philip

The former long-distance runner, from Dundee, directed her concern to politicians during an event in the Scottish Parliament.

She said little has changed since she was young.

'I still coach kids who are paying £3 to get into a track that has very bad lighting. I can't see them in the winter time. There's only one toilet. There's no drinks available,' she pointed out.

'It's quite sad that we've had so much success at the Olympics, and we've got 112 kids who all want to be like Mo Farah, and I can see that the cycle track that's just 100 metres long across the park is exactly the same, the swimming clubs are exactly the same.

'Were we prepared? No we weren't.'

'We are probably going to let down a lot of kids who are so enthused from the success that we had. Kids nowadays have got a great access to television. I didn't have that in my day. They see it and they want it.

'I feel the Government, the associations have let us down because we are not prepared to deal with all these kids that want to be the next Chris Hoy or Kat Grainger.'

Ms McColgan, who won silver in the 1988 Seoul Olympics and two golds in Commonwealth competitions, said it was lucky that the 2012 Games were a success.

Speaking as a panellist at the Festival of Politics in Holyrood, she said: 'I believe there's no legacy that I can see left in my neck of the woods. We're left to our own devices.'

In a direct plea, she said: 'I've sat on many, many panels like this and nothing happens. Everyone's got great ideas but nothing happens. Why not just listen for once and take action?'

She was joined on the panel by former Scotland rugby player John Beattie who also complained about a lack of action that would stimulate investment in sport for children.

He suggested private funding for state school sport, adding that he feels guilty about the high standards he enjoyed at private school.

'I don't think it's a Government thing alone. There's a whole corporate world that should be getting into this because there's no way you're getting more money,' he said.

'The next step to make it work would be corporate money coming into the school system to sponsor leagues, to pay teachers extra.'

The panel also included sports journalist Alison Walker and Scottish Sports Association policy director Kim Atkinson, and was chaired by Labour MSP John Park.

24 August 2012

⇨ The above information is reprinted with kind permission from *The Independent*. Please visit www.independent.co.uk for further information.

© *The Independent*

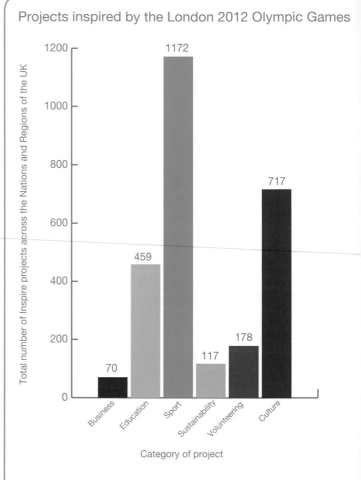

Projects inspired by the London 2012 Olympic Games

Source: Inspire Programme key facts and figures, The London Organising Committee of the Olympic Games and Paralympic Games Limited, 2012
© The London Organising Committee of the Olympic Games and Paralympic Games Limited

New findings show women run scared from outdoor exercise

Today the mental health charity Mind releases new statistics showing nine out of ten women aged over 30* battle body-confidence and low self-esteem when considering outdoor exercise.

This is leading many to take extreme measures, such as exercising when it's dark to minimise embarrassment, or to avoid outdoor activities altogether.

Outdoor exercise can be as effective as antidepressants in treating mild to moderate depression and anxiety☐and is increasingly being recognised and prescribed as a form of therapy.

However, new findings for the 'Feel better outside, feel better inside' campaign, run by Ecominds on behalf of the Big Lottery Fund, suggest that whilst many women feel unable to exercise outside confidently, they are missing fantastic opportunities to boost and maintain positive mental well-being.

Women are continuously confronted by health messages, advising them to get active to improve mental and physical health. The point is getting through as 98% of the 1,450 women surveyed were well aware of the research.

However the issue is more complex as inhibitions and low body-confidence create significant barriers to getting outside regularly, especially when feeling low.

Mind's research found women were more likely to eat comfort food (71%), listen to sad music (32%), spend time social networking (57%), go to bed (66%) or find a way to be alone (71%), than exercise.

The survey also revealed:

⇨ Two out of three feel conscious about their body shape when they exercise in public

⇨ Many doubt their own ability compared to others; 65% think it's unlikely they'll be able to keep up in an exercise group and almost a half feel they will look silly in front of others as a result of being uncoordinated

⇨ 60% are nervous about how their body reacts to exercise – their wobbly bits, sweating, passing wind or going red

⇨ Two out of three feel that if they joined an exercise group, other women would be unwelcoming and cliquey, with only 6% feeling they would be very likely to make new friends.

In response to these feelings, many women have taken extreme steps to reduce the risk of embarrassment:

⇨ Over 50% said they exercised very early in the morning or late at night solely to avoid being seen by others

⇨ Almost two out of three of women choose to exercise in a location where they're unlikely to bump into anyone they know

⇨ Over 50% don't leave the home when exercising, so as not to be seen in public – even though exercising outside is more effective for lifting mood than inside

⇨ 67% wear baggy clothing when exercising in order to hide their figure.

Beth Murphy, head of information at Mind, said:

'We all know that walking, cycling, even gardening are good for our mental health;

however, for many of us exercising in the great outdoors can be incredibly daunting, especially if already feeling low and self-confidence is at rock bottom.

'At these times you can feel like the only person in the world experiencing this, but Mind's research highlights that far from being alone, 90% of women are in exactly the same boat.

'It's time we start talking about how exercise makes us feel. We urge women to take the first step, invite a friend on a nature date and begin to support each other in taking care of our mental well-being.

Sarah,** age 37, who has experienced severe depression said:

'I have been taking anti-depressants since last February, but honestly feel that exercise has a more noticeable effect than the drugs.

'I can't believe I am saying this, but discovering outdoor exercise changed everything. I was petrified, I knew I would sweat, go red, have trouble keeping up and that everyone else in the group would be super fit. I was so incredibly scared and thought I'd be humiliated.

'However – the other people in the group were all normal – all different shapes and sizes – and no one cared what you looked like or did.

'It was the most liberating experience ever My initial reason for exercising was to lose some weight, but from that first session I realised just how good it could be for my state of mind. From there my confidence grew.'

As part of the Ecominds 'Feel better outside, feel better inside' campaign, Mind is calling for women to start talking openly about outdoor exercise, to take the first step and ask a friend to join them in an outdoor activity by sending a nature date invite at www.mind.org.uk/naturedate.

*** *Research taken from a poll of 1,450 people conducted via Survey Monkey between 13 March and 3 April 2012.*

*** *The case-study's name has been changed to protect her anonymity*

1. *Halliwell E. (2005). Up and Running? Exercise Therapy and the treatment of mild to moderate depression in primary care, Mental Health Foundation, London*

23 April 2012

⇨ The above information is reprinted with kind permission from Mind. Please visit www.mind.org.uk for further information.

Notes

⇨ Research taken from a poll of 1,450 people conducted via Survey Monkey between 13 March and 3 April 2012

⇨ Mind spokesperson and case study interviews available upon request

⇨ For more information please contact the Mind media team on T: 020 8522 1743 M: 07850 788514 E: c.swain@mind.org.uk ISDN line available: 020 8221 0817

Ecominds

⇨ Ecominds is a £7.5 million funding scheme run by Mind on behalf of the Big Lottery Fund. It funds environmental projects that help people with experience of mental distress get involved in local green activities to improve confidence, self-esteem and physical health. A total of £7.5 million has been distributed to 130 new and existing projects across England.

⇨ The 'Feel better outside, feel better inside' campaign supports Mind's lottery-funded Ecominds scheme. The campaign aims to increase public awareness of, and participation in, outdoor activities in natural environments to improve mental and physical well-being. www.mind.org.uk/ecominds

Mind

⇨ We're Mind, the mental health charity. We provide advice and support to empower anyone experiencing a mental health problem. We campaign to improve services, raise awareness and promote understanding. We won't give up until everyone experiencing a mental health problem gets both support and respect. www.mind.org.uk

Big Lottery Fund

⇨ The Big Lottery Fund's Changing Spaces programme was launched in November 2005 to help communities enjoy and improve their local environments. The programme is funding a range of activities from local food schemes and farmers markets, to education projects teaching people about the environment. Mind was awarded £8.8 million as a Changing Spaces award partner, to run its Ecominds scheme. Full details of the work of the Big Lottery Fund, its programmes and awards are available on the website: www.biglotteryfund.org.uk

Half of people in UK cannot run 100 metres

New research by YouGov for Slimming World shows nearly half of adults cannot run 100 metres.

It's likely that Usain Bolt will run the distance in less than ten seconds this weekend, but a survey has found that nearly half of adults in the UK (45%) believe it would be difficult or impossible to run 100 metres without stopping.

The online survey of 2,065 people which asked about people's weight, eating habits and fitness levels, was conducted to mark the start of Slimming World's 'Miles for Smiles' activity programme to encourage people to become more active while raising money for the NSPCC at the same time.

⇨ The survey found that women are almost twice as likely as men to be brought out in a cold sweat by the idea of running 100 metres, with 56% of women believing it would be difficult or impossible to run the distance compared to 31% of men.

⇨ When it was announced that the Olympics were to be held in London it was hoped that it would leave a legacy of a more active Britain, but the survey revealed that three out of four people (75%) in the UK never take part in competitive activity and more than half (55 %) never take part in non-competitive activity either.

⇨ In contrast, six out of ten men (59%) enjoy watching sport on TV at least once a week, with that figure likely to have risen during the Olympic season.

'These findings show how daunting the idea of physical activity can be for the many of us who lead completely sedentary lives,' says Carolyn Pallister, Slimming World's public health manager.

'It's easy to fall out of the habit of being active and the longer we go without doing it the less confident we feel. For people who are worried about their weight or poor fitness – and that's the majority of the population – the thought of taking those first steps to a more active lifestyle can feel terrifying and, with busy lives, it's easy to make excuses and decide that now just isn't the right time to make a change.

Pallister said she hoped that with the rise in sport spectators in London's 2012 Olympic Games, there will also be a rise in physical activity; however, she does concede that watching world class athletes could make people feel less capable of being active themselves.

'The real focus of any programme designed to help people become more active needs to be about helping people to build their confidence in their ability to make changes,' she said. 'Being encouraged to start slowly and find ways of being active that they enjoy and can build into their everyday life can help take the threat out of activity.

At Slimming World they find that by helping our members identify ways of moving more and supporting them to increase their activity levels gradually, they can be helped to grow their confidence as they build up to a more active lifestyle.

'Whether it's taking the stairs instead of the lift, swapping sedentary video consoles for active gaming like the Nintendo Wii or Xbox Kinect or trading nights in front of the TV for more active pursuits like taking a brisk walk, joining a zumba class or kicking a football around in the park, we see firsthand what a difference small, enjoyable changes can make.'

6 August 2012

⇨ The above information is reprinted with kind permission from YouGov. Please visit www.yougov.co.uk for further information.

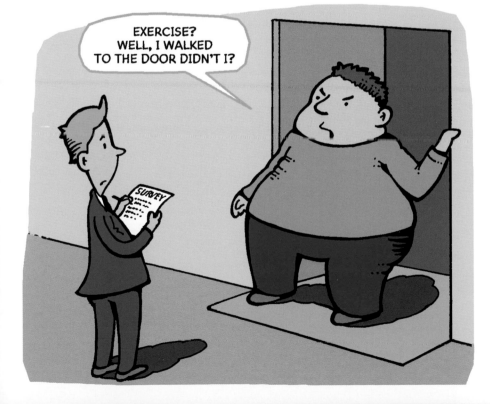

Obesity

Chapter 2

Obesity in adults

If you are obese or overweight, you have an increased risk of developing various health problems. Even a modest amount of weight loss can help to reduce your increased health risks. The best chance of losing weight, and keeping the weight off, is to be committed to a change in lifestyle. This includes eating a healthy diet and doing some regular physical activity.

Are you obese or overweight?

If you are obese or overweight, this means that you are carrying excess body fat. Being overweight or obese is not just about how you look. Over time, it means that you have an increased risk of developing various health problems. As an adult, you can find out whether you are overweight or obese and whether your health may be at risk, by calculating your body mass index (BMI) and measuring your waist circumference.

Body mass index – BMI

People are different heights and builds, so just weighing yourself cannot be used to decide if your weight is healthy. BMI is used by healthcare professionals to assess if someone's weight is putting their health at risk. It is a measure of your weight related to your height.

To calculate your BMI, you divide your weight (in kilograms) by the square of your height (in metres).

So, for example, if you weigh 70 kg and are 1.75 metres tall, your BMI is 70/(1.75 x 1.75), which is 22.9.

If you do not have scales at home, your practice nurse can measure your height, weigh you, and calculate your BMI. There are also various BMI calculators available on the Internet. For example, go to: www.eatwell.gov.uk/healthydiet/healthyweight/bmicalculator/

The table below shows how to interpret your BMI. In general, the more your BMI is over 25, the more overweight or obese you are and the greater the risk to your health.

On the whole, BMI is a good estimate of how much of your body is made up of fat. However, BMI may be less accurate in very muscular people. This is because muscle weighs heavier than fat. So, someone who is very muscular may have a relatively high BMI due to the weight of their muscle bulk but actually have a proportionally low and healthy amount of body fat.

Waist circumference

If you are overweight, measuring your waist circumference can also give some information about your risk of developing health problems (particularly coronary heart disease and type 2 diabetes). If two overweight or obese people have the same BMI, the person with a bigger waist circumference will be at a greater risk of developing health problems due to their weight. This is because it is not just whether you are carrying excess fat but where you are carrying it. The risks to your health are greater if you mainly carry a lot of extra fat around your waist ('apple-shaped'), rather than mainly on your hips and thighs ('pear-shaped').

The easiest way to measure your waist circumference is to place the tape measure around your waist at belly button level.

As a rule for a man:

⇨ If you have a waist measurement of 94 cm or above, the risk to your health is increased.

⇨ If you have a waist measurement of 102 cm or above, the risk is even higher.

As a rule for a woman:

⇨ If you have a waist measurement of 80 cm or above, the risk to your health is increased.

⇨ If you have a waist measurement of 88 cm or above, the risk is even higher.

BMI	Classed as	Health risk
Less than 18.5	Underweight	Some health risk
18.5 to 24.9	Ideal	Normal
25 to 29.9	Overweight	Moderate health risk
30 to 39.9	Obese	High health risk
40 and over	Very obese	Very high health risk

Note: for people from Asian backgrounds, the increased health risks may start at a lower waist circumference. Your doctor or practice nurse can advise.

What are the health risks of being overweight or obese?

If you are overweight or obese, from day to day you may:

⇨ Feel tired and lacking in energy.

⇨ Experience breathing problems (for example, shortness of breath when moving around, or not being able to cope with sudden bursts of physical activity like running across the road).

⇨ Feel that you sweat a lot compared with other people.

⇨ Develop skin irritation.

⇨ Have difficulty sleeping.

⇨ Get complaints from your partner that you snore.

⇨ Experience back and joint pains which can affect your mobility.

You may also have an increased risk of developing:

⇨ Impaired glucose tolerance (pre-diabetes).

⇨ Type 2 diabetes.

⇨ High cholesterol or triglyceride levels.

⇨ High blood pressure.

⇨ Coronary heart disease.

⇨ Stroke.

⇨ Sleep apnoea (this is when your breathing patterns are disturbed while you are sleeping, due to excess weight around your chest, neck and airways).

⇨ Fertility problems.

⇨ Complications in pregnancy (including an increased risk of high blood pressure during pregnancy, diabetes during pregnancy, preterm labour, Caesarean section).

⇨ Stress incontinence (leaking urine when you are, for example, laughing, coughing, etc.).

⇨ Gallstones.

⇨ Cancers (including colon, breast and endometrial (womb) cancer).

⇨ Gout.

⇨ Fatty liver.

Many people can also develop psychological problems because of being overweight or obese. For example: low self-esteem; poor self-image (not liking how you look); low confidence; feelings of isolation. These feelings may affect your relationships with family members and friends and, if they become severe, may lead to depression.

Being obese (having a BMI >30) can also affect your overall life expectancy: you are more likely to die at a younger age. An analysis in 2009 of almost one million people from around the world showed that if you have a BMI between 30 and 35, you are likely to die two to four years earlier than average. If your BMI is between 40 to 45, you are likely to die eight to ten years earlier than average.

Another analysis showed that if you are a woman who is obese at the age of 40, you are likely to die 7.1 years earlier than average. If you are a man who is obese at the age of 40, you are likely to die 5.8 years earlier than average. If you smoke as well, your life expectancy is reduced even further.

How common is it to obese or overweight?

In the UK:

⇨ Between six and seven out of ten men have a BMI >25 and so are overweight or obese.

⇨ Between five and six out of ten women have a BMI >25 and so are overweight or obese.

⇨ Around one in four men and one in four women in the UK have a BMI >30 and so are obese.

⇨ Around two in 100 adults are severely (also called morbidly) obese (BMI >40).

The number of obese people in the UK is rising, particularly among young adults. Since 1980, the number of obese adults in the UK has nearly tripled. This has been called the obesity epidemic.

What are the causes of being overweight or obese?

In some respects, the cause sounds quite simple. Your weight depends on how much energy you take in (the calories in food and drink) and how much energy your body uses (burns) up:

⇨ If the amount of calories that you eat equals the amount of energy that your body uses up, then your weight remains stable.

⇨ If you eat more calories than you burn up, you put on weight. The excess energy is converted into fat and stored in your body.

⇨ If you eat fewer calories than you burn up, you lose weight. Your body has to tap into its fat stores to get the extra energy it needs.

A common wrong belief is to think that if you are overweight or obese, you have a low metabolic rate. (Your metabolic rate or metabolism is the amount of energy that your body needs to keep going.) In fact, if you are obese or overweight you have a normal, or even high, metabolic rate (as you use up more energy carrying the extra weight).

The reasons why energy taken in may not balance energy used up, and may lead to weight gain, include the following.

How much you eat and drink

Most people in the UK live where tasty food can be found at almost any time of day or night. Many of the foods that people eat are those higher in calories (particularly fatty and sugary foods), so-called energy-dense foods. Although your body gives you a feeling of fullness after eating enough (satiety), you can easily ignore this feeling if you are enjoying tasty foods. Food portion sizes in general have increased. There has also been a tendency to eat out more over recent years. If you eat out, you are more likely to eat food that is more energy-dense than you would eat at home. The amount of processed foods and ready-made meals available has also increased in response to our busy lives. These are often foods that are more energy-dense as well. However, even healthy foods contain calories and can tip the energy balance if we eat too much of them.

What you drink is also important. Alcohol and sugary drinks contain a lot of calories. Even fresh fruit juices that you may think are healthy can make up a significant part of your daily calorie intake if you drink too much of them.

In short, many people are overweight or obese simply because they eat and drink more than their body needs.

Your physical activity levels

Where does physical activity fit in to your current lifestyle? Most people in the UK do not do enough physical activity. Fewer people these days have jobs which are energetic. The variety of labour-saving devices and gadgets in most homes, and the overuse of cars, means that most people end up using up much less energy compared with previous generations. The average person in the UK watches 26 hours of television per week, and many even more (the couch potato syndrome).

A lack of physical activity by many people is thought to be a major cause of the increase in obesity in recent years.

Genetics

You are more likely to be obese if one of your parents is obese, or both of your parents are obese. This may partly be due to learning bad eating habits from your parents. But, some people actually inherit a tendency in their genes that makes them prone to overeat. So, for some people, part of the problem is genetic.

It is not fully understood how this genetic factor works. It has something to do with the control of appetite. When you eat, certain hormones and brain chemicals send messages to parts of your brain to say that you have had enough, and to stop eating. In some people, this control of appetite and the feeling of fullness (satiety) may be faulty, or not as good as it is in others.

However, if you do inherit a tendency to overeat, it is not inevitable that you will become overweight or obese. You can learn about the power of your appetite, ways to resist it, be strict on what you eat, and do some regular physical activity. But you are likely to struggle more than most people where your weight is concerned. You may find it more difficult to stop yourself from gaining weight or to lose weight.

Medical problems

Less than one in 100 obese people has a 'medical' cause for their obesity. For example, conditions such as Cushing's syndrome and an underactive thyroid are rare causes of weight gain. Women with polycystic ovary syndrome may also be overweight.

Some medicines such as steroids, some antidepressants, sulphonylureas and sodium valproate may contribute to weight gain. If you give up smoking, your appetite may increase and, as a result, you may put on weight. People with low mood or depression may also have a tendency to eat more energy-dense 'comfort' foods and so gain weight.

25 August 2011

Original author: Dr Tim Kenny. Current version: Dr Michelle Wright.

⇨ The above information is reprinted with kind permission from Patient, part of Egton Medical Information Systems Limited (EMIS). Please visit www.patient.co.uk for further information.

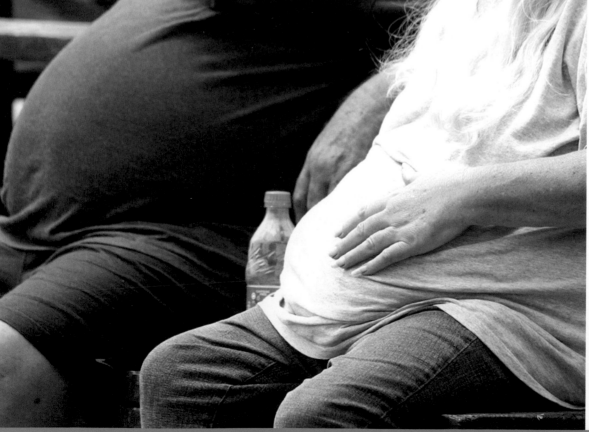

Fat but fit: obese people can be healthy and in good metabolic shape

A new research study has found that people who are considered obese can actually be in good health and are no more likely to suffer from poor health as a result of their weight – in fact, over 40% of obese people could actually be metabolically healthy and fit.

By Christopher Hughes

Defining obesity

It is well known that obesity, or simply being overweight, can lead to a number of serious health-related problems. Some of these include heart disease, high blood pressure, aching joints and even cancer. But how do doctors determine whether someone is a 'healthy' weight, overweight or obese? Well they use what is called the body mass index, or BMI for short, and they calculate this using a person's weight and height. People with a BMI of 25 or more are considered overweight while those with a BMI of over 30 are obese. To get more accurate results they also measured the body fat percentage of people using skin fold calipers. For men, a body fat percentage less than 25 is normal and anything over is considered obese – for women that cut off stands at 30.

What does the new study say?

But it's not all black and white. This new study found that some obese people, people with a BMI over 30, are actually 'metabolically healthy'. This means that they don't show any of the usual health problems associated with their weight, like diabetes, high cholesterol and high blood sugar levels. This 'metabolically healthy' group also had higher levels of fitness, based on heart and lung performance, than other extremely overweight people.

The researchers also wanted to discover if these 'metabolically fit' people were less likely to develop health problems, or die from these problems, than the less 'metabolically healthy' obese people and people of normal weight. To do this the researchers conducted the largest ever study on the subject by examining over 43,000 people in America between 1979 and 2003. They measured the BMI, body fat percentage and overall level of fitness of the participants and recorded how many became ill with health problems and also how many died because of their weight.

The study concluded that 46% of obese people were actually 'metabolically healthy', meaning that they had the same mortality risk for heart disease or cancer that people of normal weight have. Based on a number of cardiovascular tests, including running on a treadmill, this group of 46% were actually fitter than other obese people. The lead author of the study, Dr Francisco Ortega, added that 'obesity is associated with a large number of chronic diseases such as heart disease and cancer... there is a group of obese people that do not suffer the metabolic complications associated with obesity'.

The researchers discovered that the 'metabolically healthy' group of obese people had a 38% lower risk of early death than their unhealthy obese peers. There is no difference in the healthy obese people and the healthy normal weight people, researchers said. After adjusting for several other factors, including age, gender and whether people smoked or not, they also found that these healthy obese people, when compared to the unhealthy obese people, were:

⇨ 44% less likely to die from heart disease.

⇨ 32% less likely to die from cancer.

⇨ 51% less likely to suffer a heart attack or have a stroke.

The researchers tried to be as accurate as possible by having the participants fill out a detailed questionnaire, including information on their medical and lifestyle history. Blood pressure, cholesterol and blood sugar levels were also measured to ensure accurate findings.

How does this affect me?

The study concluded that regardless of body weight or fat, people with better aerobic fitness have a lower risk for heart disease, cancer and even death. The study has had a great affect on how doctors can now treat overweight and obese patients. Dr Ortega has advised that 'physicians could assess fitness, fatness and metabolic markers to do a better estimation of the risk of cardiovascular disease and cancer of obese patients'.

However, it's still important to remember that obesity can still increase your risk of developing other health-related problems such as joint pain, back pain and even sleeping problems. If you are overweight or obese, this research highlights the importance of regular exercise no matter how much you weigh.

Source:

Ortega, F.B., Lee, D.C., Katzmarzyk, P.T., Ruiz, J.R., Sui, X., Church, T.S. and Blair S.N. 2012. The intriguing metabolically healthy but obese phenotype: cardiovascular prognosis and role of fitness, European Heart Journal, published online 4 September 2012.

6 December 2012

⇨ The above article is printed with kind permission from the author Christopher Hughes.

The true financial cost of obesity

Within ten years, 40% of the population could be obese, requiring billions in health spending.

By Professor Tony Leeds

GPs and surgeons yesterday launched a campaign to combat obesity, saying current strategies were not working.

Around 30,000 Britons die prematurely each year of obesity-related conditions, and many more cope day-to-day with conditions including heart disease, diabetes and osteoarthritis.

But attached to this appalling human cost is a financial one, and it's snowballing. For every month of inaction now, the cost will multiply, to the point where – in ten years – it could double.

Today's situation is grim enough. Almost a quarter of adults in England are obese (with a body mass index (BMI) of 30 or over). Around 800,000 are 'morbidly obese' – with a BMI of 40 or higher, the level at which life insurance companies may decline cover. In short, we are moving towards a situation where a million Britons' lives are threatened daily. Again, a truly awful situation in human terms alone.

But what are the financial costs, and why should politicians act now?

An oft-quoted Foresight report predicted that the direct economic costs of overweight and obesity would be £6.4 billion a year by 2015.

But it put the wider costs of elevated BMI – e.g. related conditions as well as impact on the economy through sickness and absence, etc. – at a massive £27 billion by the same time.

The costs of effective treatment are rising: for bariatric surgery it is around £32.3 million per annum.

Look deeper at this single area of bariatric surgery. Just how many people would qualify for surgery right now and what would it cost if they all wanted it?

Guidance from the Government's National Institute for Health and Clinical Excellence (NICE) sets the surgery threshold at a BMI of 40, or 35 if they have a related health complication like diabetes.

Clearly not everyone who is eligible for surgery will get it as not everyone is medically suitable, not everyone wants surgery, and individual primary care trusts apply their own criteria.

But the point here is that, if everyone who qualified actually had it, the cost to the NHS in the first year alone could jump from £32.3 million per annum, to £9.1 billion.

So the cost of obesity is already into the realms of billions of pounds, but potential solutions will cost billions too. This is a point at which alarm bells should start ringing.

How it could unfold

The long-term trend in obesity prevalence has been relentlessly upwards. It may now be flattening off, but the prevalence of obesity-related conditions is still rising, reflecting the delayed effect of obesity on the body's metabolism and mechanics.

There are also alarming signs of rising obesity in children too.

So how could Britain look ten years from now? Well, if our leaders don't grasp the nettle, here are some predictions:

⇨ 35-40 per cent of the population could be obese

⇨ There could be a 100 per cent increase in knee replacement surgery, and a doubling of annual costs, to £1,500 million (based on £803 million costs in 2009/10 and 29% rise in four years)

⇨ The number of people with diabetes could soar by 40 per cent, with a doubling of their medication bill, to £1,400 million

⇨ Costs of treating high blood pressure could rise further. The three-fold increase in GP prescriptions for anti-hypertensives from 2000 to 2010 reflected better and more effective treatment of high blood pressure. A likely further rise over the next ten years could perhaps be attenuated by effective obesity management.

Speculation? Yes. But the figures are not beyond the bounds of possibility.

GPs hold the key to this spiralling situation. They could improve and save lives – and money – right now.

But they need two things.

Firstly, they need training in weight management – ironically, most GPs acknowledge that they have no specialist knowledge of the one subject which causes so many patient problems. If proper training was available, every local surgery could have an 'obesity GP', with a strategy to drive down weight, and drive up health.

And secondly, GPs need to be able to offer patients more practical help.

At the moment, GPs can offer four options – 'a healthy diet'; a community-based diet programme; a single drug therapy; or gastric surgery.

While the first three are fine for those who are modestly overweight, heavier patients could take many years to lose the weight, and in most cases, this is just not going to happen.

And yet at the other end of the scale, while the cost of surgery is proven to be recovered in three years through savings on diabetic drug costs, surgery cannot possibly be provided to everyone who might benefit. And it is, quite rightly, viewed by many as a last resort.

By far the greatest need for weight loss is in the 'middle ground' of around three stone but there is a 'therapeutic void' in the middle ground where we have little to offer. If patients could lose two to three stone quickly, and maintain the weight loss, millions could be freed from miserable health conditions and expensive medication. And, vitally, it would halt the escalation of their obesity, which would otherwise lead to even greater problems.

Diet can in fact address the needs in this middle ground. A clinical trial, published in the *British Medical Journal*, demonstrated that three quarters of patients with sleep apnoea – the hidden killer – could be helped, while another showed how people with disabling osteoarthritis could lose weight, become more mobile and escape from social isolation at home.

I now declare an interest: I am in the privileged position of combining NHS practice with work within the private sector that includes commissioning research. I have been able to encourage key clinical scientists to undertake the clinical trials needed to demonstrate how effective weight loss and maintenance of one to two stone with formula diet can give sustained health benefits. I have also been able to use formula diet in NHS practice thereby developing a model for how this can be done in an ordinary clinical setting.

Surely it's time for this Government – with its openness towards the private sector – to recognise that modern, safe, evidence-based, low-cost, diet solutions are now available, and actively encourage GPs to treat and manage obesity.

Professor Tony Leeds is a physician with a specialist interest in obesity at Central Middlesex and Whittington hospitals, London, and medical director of Cambridge Weight Plan.

The opinions in politics.co.uk's Comment and Analysis section are those of the author and are no reflection of the views of the website or its owners.

16 April 2012

⇨ The above information is reprinted with kind permission from Politics.co.uk. Please visit www. politics.co.uk for further information.

Childhood obesity

Information from Royal College of Paediatrics and Child Health.

What do we know?

Nearly a third (31%) of children aged two to 15 are overweight or obese.[1] The direct cost of obesity to the NHS is estimated to be £4.2 billion a year.[2] The causes of obesity are complex, but the problem is closely linked with obesogenic environments, which encourage children to consume too much food that is rich in salt, fat and sugar and encourage a sedentary lifestyle. Parents need more support to help their children to maintain a healthy weight. Overweight parents often have overweight children, and perinatal programming and their lifestyle choices have a significant influence.[3] Parenting style has an impact on children's lifestyle and emotional well-being, with a subsequent impact on weight. The consequences of obesity later in life include problems with joints and bones, hypertension, heart failure, high blood pressure and high levels of blood fats. Increasingly, teenagers are developing early onset type 2 diabetes as a result of their weight. Obesity can also have psychological effects on children's self-esteem. Although recent years have seen a levelling-off of the rapid rise in childhood obesity, there is little cause for complacency on the issue.

What can we do?

Prevention and treatment of obesity depends on all levels of society and government taking action – from health professionals, in educating teachers, parents and children themselves, regulating and working with the food manufacturing industry, and using fiscal measures where appropriate. This has the objective of achieving the cultural shift in improved nutrition and increased exercise to achieve a sustained decrease in the numbers of children that are overweight or obese.

Health professionals

The management of children with weight problems needs to be sensitively addressed, and therefore all health professionals should receive training on the issues.[4] NICE (clinical guidance 43) reminds those working with children that treatment 'may stigmatise them and put them at risk of bullying... Confidentiality and building self-esteem are particularly important if help is offered at school.'[5] These principles of discretion and sensitivity are particularly applicable to the National Child Measurement Programme, which offers an opportunity for health professionals to engage with parents and their children where the latter's weight is cause for concern.

Parents, carers and schools

Parents need to be supported and encouraged to be role models for their children; health professionals should emphasise the importance of parental lifestyles and parenting style when their children's weight is considered. The role of those who engage with children on a day-to-day basis has a key influence on whether the child maintains a healthy lifestyle. A number of studies demonstrate a link between parents' diets, physical activity and their children's own relationship with food and exercise habits.[6]

Breastfeeding[7] also appears to have a small but consistent reductive impact on childhood obesity.[8]

When children are in education, high-quality school dinners can ensure that children eat at least one nutritious meal a day. Nutritional standards have been introduced in English primary (since 2007) and secondary (since 2008) schools,[9] with similar initiatives in the Hungry

for Success programme leading to legislation in Scotland,[10] Appetite for Life in Wales[11] and Catering for Healthier Lifestyles in Northern Ireland.[12] However, the introduction of free schools and academies in England which need not comply with central requirements, means these standards may be breached by new organisations. A systematic study of pupils' behaviour and concentration in six Sheffield schools of 146 children aged eight to ten over a 12-week period by the Schools Food Trust found a positive correlation with school meals provision.[13] Universal provision of school meals would also ensure that all children receive a healthy meal at least once every day, and is a successful feature of the Swedish education system.[14] The estimated costs of such provision in England would be £1,068 million in primary and £816 million in secondary schools.[15]

Levels of physical exercise also have a significant influence on obesity development. A 2011 joint report by the four nations' Chief Medical Officers made recommendations about increasing the population's activity levels and for the first time included recommendations for the early years, stating that children and young people over five years old should exercise for at least 60 minutes at moderate intensity, while those under five should maintain at least 180 minutes physical activity, spread throughout the day.[16] Encouraging active travel and play should be a

priority for local authorities, using Health and Wellbeing Boards as a conduit for planning appropriate action. This action might include looking at traffic-calming measures to make areas safer to play, ensuring public spaces can be reached by foot and by bicycle, and identifying and addressing existing barriers that mitigate against children walking and cycling.[17]

The food industry

Only a ban on advertising before the 9pm 'watershed' would prevent children from viewing unhealthy content during family orientated programming. In 2007, restrictions on 'junk food' advertising during programmes specifically targeted at children were introduced. However, OfCom, the broadcast regulator, found that this only reduced exposure to advertising of unhealthy food for children by 37%, and for older children (ten to 15-year-olds) only 22%.[18] Children of all ages are still exposed to a large amount of unhealthy food and drink advertising via popular all-ages programmes, such as soaps or reality shows. Research suggests that younger children are unable to distinguish between advertisements and other content,[19] consequently normalising these products into the mainstream diet of children.[20]

While parents and those that care for children have a role to play in the food that their children consume, the food manufacturing industry have a major influence in terms of marketing and pricing. Although the Government's public health responsibility deal has made some progress, with manufacturers reducing salt and sugar, RCPCH believes that more stringent controls of food manufacturing and marketing would be beneficial for children's health.

Fiscal measures

Research suggests that increasing tax on unhealthy food and drink results in reduced calorific intake.[21] This is an effective and cost-saving policy: an Australian study calculated

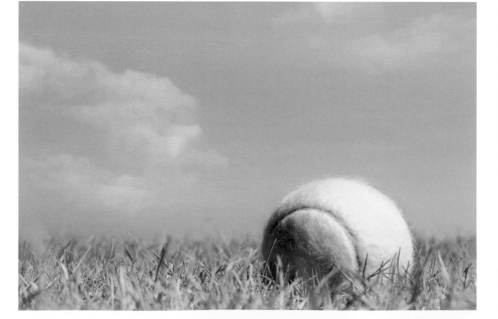

an impressive saving of 559,000 disability-adjusted life-years (DALYs) on a 10% tax, with only AU$18 million investment.[22] Hungary and Denmark have recently introduced so-called 'fat taxes'. When the policy has been mooted previously, it has been suggested that the policy might be regressive (i.e. affecting the poor disproportionately), although similar arguments have been made around alcohol minimum pricing, with the rejoinder that

'[t]here may also be concerns that the impact of minimum pricing would be regressive but the harms from alcohol also appear to affect lower social groups',[23] The same could be said of obesity, particularly with the socioeconomic gradient of childhood obesity (at Reception year, 12.6% of children in the poorest decile are obese, compared to 6.8% in the most affluent decile).[24]

Recommendations

The RCPCH recommends action in four areas, with the intention of achieving a cultural shift to reduce the numbers of our children and young people that are obese or overweight:

⇨ All health professionals should be trained in weight management issues, following NICE and SIGN[25] guidance, alongside emphasising the importance of parenting style and parents' lifestyles when their children's weight is considered.

⇨ The extension of free school meals so that it is universal should be looked at and costed, while academies and free schools should be mandated to follow nutritional standards.

⇨ Local authorities need to implement strategies to encourage active travel and play, by making the built environment more accessible for young pedestrians and cyclists. These plans can be implemented through joint partnership with Health and Wellbeing Boards.

⇨ Food manufacturers' influence on younger children should be curtailed by implementing a ban on 'junk' food advertising before the 9pm watershed.

⇨ Increases in taxation on foods high in salt, sugar and fat in other countries should be independently evaluated, scoped and costed with a view to implementation across the UK.

April 2012

⇨ Information from the Royal College of Paediatrics and Child Health. Please visit www.rcpch. ac.uk for further information.

References

1. Health and Social Care Information Centre (2009), Children's overweight and obesity prevalence, by survey year, age-group and sex http://www.ic.nhs.uk/webfiles/publications/HSE/Health_Survey_for_England_1995_to_1997_Revised_Childrens%20Table%204.xls

2. Department of Health, Obesity: General Information http://www.dh.gov.uk/en/Publichealth/Obesity/DH_078098 accessed 29 September 2011

3. Whitaker RC, Wright JA, Pepe MS, Seidel KD, Dietz WH (1997), 'Predicting obesity in young adulthood from childhood and parental obesity', N Engl J Med. 337:869–873

4. Royal College of Physicians (2010), The training of health professionals for the prevention and treatment of overweight and obesity

5. National Institute for Health and Clinical Excellence (2006), CG043: Obesity: guidance on the prevention, identification, assessment and management of overweight and obesity in adults and children

6. Rudolf, M (2009), Tackling obesity through the Healthy Child Programme

7. RCPCH 'Breastfeeding position statement' (2011)

8. S Arenz, R Rücker, B Koletzko and R von Kries (2004), 'Breast-feeding and childhood obesity – a systematic review', International Journal of Obesity 28:1247–1256

9. Parliamentary Office of Science and Technology (2009), Nutritional standards in UK schools

10. Schools (Health Promotion and Nutrition) (Scotland) Act 2007 (http://scotland.gov.uk/Topics/Education/Schools/HLivi/foodnutrition) and the Nutritional Requirements for Food and Drink in Schools (Scotland) Regulations 2008 (http://scotland.gov.uk/Publications/2008/09/12090355/0) http://scotland.gov.uk/Topics/Education/Schools/HLivi/schoolmeals

11. Appetite for Life http://wales.gov.uk/topics/educationandskills/schoolshome/foodanddrink/appetiteforlife/?skip=1&lang=en

12. Department for Education (2001), Catering for Healthier Lifestyles: Compulsory Nutritional Standards for School Meals, http://www.deni.gov.uk/catering_for_healthier_lifestyles-2.pdf

13. School Food Trust (2009), School lunch and behaviour: systematic observation of classroom behaviour following a school dining room intervention http://www.schoolfoodtrust.org.uk/UploadDocs/Library/Documents/sl&b3findings.pdf

14. Hodgson, S (2010), Free school meals lift children out of poverty, accessed 9 November 2011 http://www.epolitix.com/latestnews/article-detail/newsarticle/free-school-meals-lift-children-out-of-poverty/

15. Parliamentary Office of Science and Technology (2009), Nutritional standards in UK schools

16. Department of Health (2011), At least five a week: Evidence on the impact of physical activity and its relationship to health – A report from the Chief Medical Officer

17. Sustrans (2009), Information sheet FH13: Active play and travel

18. Ofcom (2010), HFSS advertising restrictions – Final review, accessed 9 November 2011 http://stakeholders.ofcom.org.uk/market-data-research/tv-research/hfss-final-review/

19. Young B (2003), 'Does food advertising influence children's food choices?', International Journal of Advertising 22: 441-459

20. British Heart Foundation (2011), Unhealthy food and drink marketing to children, accessed 9 November 2011 http://www.bhf.org.uk/publications/view-publication.aspx?ps=1001659

21. L Epstein, K Dearing, L Roba1, E Finkelstein (2010), 'The Influence of Taxes and Subsidies on Energy Purchased in an Experimental Purchasing Study', Psychological Science 21(3):406-414

22. G Sacks, J L Veerman, M Moodie and B Swinburn (2011), ''Traffic light' nutrition labelling and 'junk-food' tax: a modelled comparison of cost-effectiveness for obesity prevention', International Journal of Obesity 35: 1001-1009

23. Ludbrook, A (2009), 'Minimum pricing of alcohol', Health Economics 18(12): 1357-60

24. National Obesity Observatory (2011), Prevalence of obesity by deprivation decile: Children in Reception and Year 6 (National Child Measurement Programme 2009/10) http://www.noo.org.uk/uploads/doc/vid_11475_Slides_child.ppt

25. Scottish Intercollegiate Guidelines Network (2010), Management of Obesity, A national clinical guideline

New UK obesity centre offers surgery to teens

London hospital says treatment is necessary to fight epidemic among children.

By Sanchez Manning

A London hospital has set up the United Kingdom's first specialist centre offering extreme weight loss surgery for children and teenagers.

Childhood obesity rates are rising fast in the UK, with latest statistics showing that a third of children aged ten to 11 in England suffer from obesity or weight issues.

'Childhood obesity rates are rising fast in the UK.'

In Southwark, the south London borough where Britain's first paediatric bariatric (weight-loss) surgery service is located, 40 per cent of secondary school children are classed as obese or overweight.

Ashish Desai, the surgeon who decided to set up the new centre at King's College Hospital to cater for 13- to 18-year-olds, said it was in response to what is becoming an epidemic. So far he has performed drastic weight loss procedures, mostly gastric band operations, on four teenagers.

Increasing numbers of young people in the United Kingdom are having bariatric surgery procedures that are normally carried out on adults. The National Obesity Forum estimates that up to 30 youngsters a year are travelling abroad with their parents for such treatment.

Such is the demand that hospitals in Sheffield, Leeds, Nottingham, Oxford, Cardiff and Newcastle are believed to be planning paediatric bariatric centres.

The youngest patient Mr Desai has operated on was a 13-year-old boy suffering from bone problems related to his obesity that meant he had to use a wheelchair.

According to the Indian-born physician, two of the other operations he performed are already proving to be successful.

'Two of the patients who have had long-term follow-ups of two to six months say they are extremely pleased with the results,' he said. 'They say that their attitude to food has changed completely. And now rather than going for the chips and fried food they go towards the salad.'

Mr Desai said surgery can provide a lasting solution for a wide range of obesity-related problems including diabetes, sleep apnoea and bone or liver disorders.

If patients maintain a good diet and exercise regime after having the procedure, they can typically expect to lose between 30 per cent and 50 per cent of their excess body weight.

One of Mr Desai's patients, Jayne (not her real name), had gastric band surgery in February, having an elastic band across the top end of her stomach to restrict the amount of food she can eat before feeling full. At the time of the operation she was 17, weighed 23 stone and had a body mass index (BMI) of 45.

She said: 'There are things in my life that mounted up and I used food as my comfort. I tried loads of diets but my weight was a brick wall.' In the two months after the operation she lost five stone and dropped four dress sizes.

But Mr Desai warned that weight-loss surgery is by no means a quick-fix solution to shifting the pounds – it is the last resort. He emphasised that any young people who attend his service go through an intensive six-month treatment programme with a dietician, a paediatrician and a psychologist.

'A third of children aged ten to 11 in England suffer from obesity or weight issues.'

After this time patients must still meet strict criteria even to be considered for the surgery, including having a BMI of at least 40 and having reached full puberty. They must further possess the 'mental maturity' to understand the implications of the operation. 'They should understand this surgery is drastic and will require lifelong commitment and changes in diet and lifestyle,' Mr Desai said.

Another important factor is the aftercare the young people receive, with patients attending between ten and 12 follow-up appointments annually.

However, Mr Desai added: 'The main goal that the community and the Government need to work together to achieve is to stop this problem through prevention.'

13 May 2012

⇨ The above information is reprinted with kind permission from *The Independent*. Please visit www.independent.co.uk for further information.

Obese children to be put up for adoption

A couple may have their obese children removed after social services ruled they had not lost enough weight.

By Nick Collins, science correspondent

The mother and father of seven children, six of whom are overweight, face the 'unbearable' prospect of never seeing their four youngest again if authorities act on a threat to remove them.

Three girls aged 11, five and one, and a boy aged five, are to be put up for adoption or 'fostered without contact' because their parents failed to help them slim down.

This means the parents will be unable to trace them and the family could only be reunited if the children attempt to find their family when they are grown up.

Social services warned the couple three years ago that their children would be taken away from them if they did not bring their weight under control.

The family spent two years living in a special council-funded house in which they were placed under a curfew and only three of the children were permitted to live with their parents at any one time.

But although they were placed under constant supervision and social workers observed them during meal times, no dietary rules were imposed and there was no significant improvement in the children's weight.

On Tuesday social workers informed the parents, who have been married for 20 years, of their decision to permanently remove their children.

The couple, from Dundee, are not guilty of any crime and have faced no accusations of deliberate abuse or cruelty.

Critics said the case, which is without precedent in Britain, was a serious breach of the family's human rights and exposed the worrying extent to which the State can interfere in family life.

The mother, aged 42, told the *Mail on Sunday:* 'They picked on us because of our size to start with and they just haven't let go, despite the fact we've done everything to lose weight and meet their demands.'

The father, aged 56, added: 'The pressure of living in the family unit would have broken anyone. We were being treated like children and cut off from the outside world. To have a social worker stand and watch you eat is intolerable.'

A Dundee City Council spokesperson said: 'The council always acts in the best interests of children, with their welfare and safety in mind.'

5 September 2011

⇨ The above information is reprinted with kind permission from *The Telegraph*. Please visit www.telegraph.co.uk for further information.

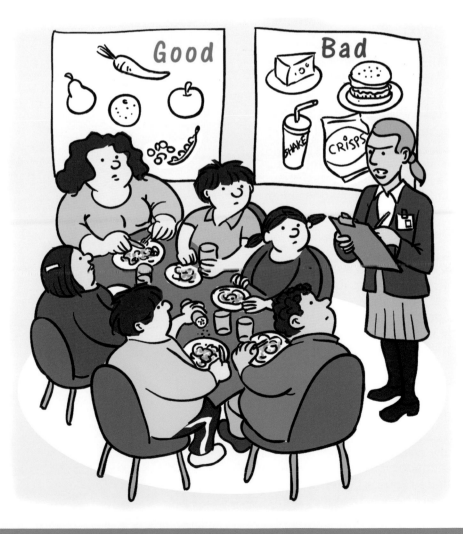

The NHS jobsworths employed to brand kids as fat

The NHS jobsworths have produced yet another set of scare statistics, this time on 'child obesity'.

By Adam Collyer

NHS figures for the past year show 19% of children in their final year of primary school were classed as obese, compared with 18.7% the previous year.

But obesity fell to 9.4% in children going into reception, down from 9.8% the previous year.

Apart from producing a great source of copy for the media, what is the use of these statistics?

They are produced by The National Child Measurement Programme (copyright: Tony Blair 1995). This measures all school kids when they start primary school and again as they get to the end of primary school.

The purpose, according to their website, is:

'The information collected helps your local NHS provider to plan and provide better health services for the children in your area.'

In other words, they serve no purpose – unless 'health services' includes putting pressure on parents to turn their kids into anorexics.

We all know that cakes and chips are bad for our kids, don't we? And we all know that feeding our kids healthy food is a good idea. The statistics prove that – wait for it – people feed their kids cake and chips anyway.

Obviously no figures are published for the cost of all this, as NHS finances are completely opaque to the public. But the cost of this measurement programme must be quite high. The survey is after all measuring a million pupils every year. The survey – even without the pseudo 'actions' that are taken as a result of it – must run into many millions of pounds of our taxes.

One can only hope that not too many children (and their parents) are made miserable by being branded 'obese' when a fifth of kids are heavier than they are.

But mostly, really, the jobsworths who waste their lives running this programme just need to be told to p*** off. We don't need their useless information, and we don't want our taxes wasted on their salaries.

They are a great example of why the NHS is crumbling.

In case you are indeed one of those jobsworths yourself reading this, and ask whether I am embittered by myself being a victim of this 1984-style programme, the answer is that no, I have not fallen foul of it myself.

14 December 2011

⇨ The above information is reprinted with kind permission from Adam Collyer. Please visit www.adamcollyer.wordpress.com for further information.

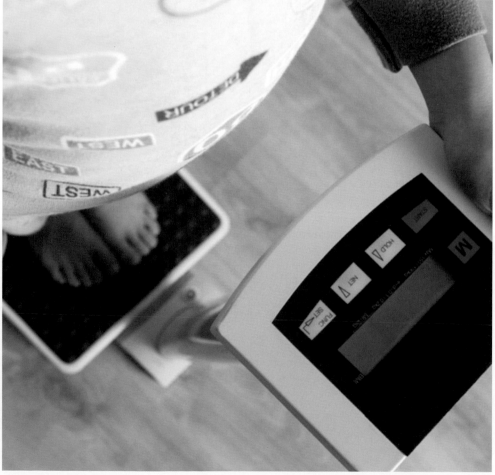

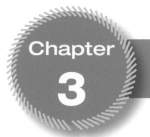

Fitness training tips

It's important to exercise safely and effectively. Robin Gargrave of YMCAfit, one of the UK's top trainers of fitness professionals, shares his tips on getting into shape safely.

When should I exercise?

There's no right time to exercise. It depends on the individual. 'You need to listen to your body,' says Robin. 'Some people feel rough in the morning, whereas others can hop out of bed and do a 10 mile run.'

Don't exercise for two to three hours after a heavy meal. If you exercise straight after a large meal, you're likely to experience nausea, stomach cramps and discomfort.

Can I have a snack before exercising?

You can have a small snack before your workout, such as a piece of fruit or a drink. Robin advises against snacks that are high in sugar, including soft drinks.

'You might get a quick energy boost but it'll probably be followed by a sudden energy slump.' Choose starchy foods, such as brown bread or bananas, which help keep your energy levels constant during exercise.

Should I warm up before exercise?

Warming up is essential before exercising. 'Without a warm-up, your workout won't be as efficient as it could

be,' says Robin. 'Your muscles won't be warm and will be less supple, which can increase your risk of injury.'

Start with slow, gentle movements, such as walking, and gradually build the intensity, such increasing your walking pace to a gentle jog.

Eight to ten minutes will warm up the muscles and get them ready for higher-intensity activity. The warm-up process sends oxygen to the muscles, where it works with glucose to produce energy, Robin says. This ensures that the body works more efficiently, and that your workout gives better results.

What is aerobic activity?

Aerobic activity is any activity where the body's large muscles move in a rhythmic manner for a continuous period of time. Also called endurance activity, it's great for improving the health of your heart and lungs. Examples include:

⇨ running

⇨ walking

⇨ cycling

⇨ swimming.

'Aerobic activity is vital for burning off calories, weight management and general health,' says Robin.

What's the importance of strength training?

Strength-training activities, such as weight lifting, involve short bursts of effort. Strength training burns calories and builds and strengthens muscle. Benefits of strength training include increasing bone density, strengthening joints, and improving balance, stability and posture.

'It increases your ability to do everyday tasks without getting so tired,' says Robin. 'The more muscle mass you have, the easier it is to burn calories, even when the body is at rest.'

Recommended physical activity levels

⇨ Children under five years old should do 180 minutes every day.

⇨ Young people (five to 18 years old) should do 60 minutes every day.

⇨ Adults (19–64 years old) should do 150 minutes every week.

⇨ Older adults (65 and over) should do 150 minutes every week.

Do I need to stretch?

Stretching helps to improve flexibility, balance and posture. To stretch properly and safely, slowly stretch the muscle just until you feel resistance. Resistance is the point at which you feel a slight pull. It should not be painful. Stop and hold each stretch for ten to 20 seconds without bouncing up and down.

During the stretch, breathe deeply and regularly. Don't hold your breath. Make sure your muscles are warmed up before you stretch. The best time to stretch is after exercise, when your muscles are most supple.

What's the importance of cooling down?

Immediately after your workout, take time to cool down. This gradually lowers your heart rate and allows your body to recover. It may help reduce muscle injury, stiffness and soreness. Walk or continue your activity at a low intensity for five to ten minutes. It's then an ideal time to stretch, and you're more likely to improve your flexibility.

Should I have a rest day?

With moderate-intensity aerobic activity, whether it's heavy gardening or cycling, you're encouraged to do a little every day. Adults should do 150 minutes (two hours and 30 minutes) of moderate-intensity aerobic activity a week. Children aged five to 18 should do 60 minutes of moderate to vigorous aerobic activity every day.

It's important to rest when you do vigorous-intensity aerobic activity, such as running. The body repairs and strengthens itself between workouts, and over-training can weaken even the strongest athletes.

What should I drink?

It's important to drink fluid during any exercise that lasts for more than 30 minutes.

Water may be enough for low-intensity exercise up to 45–50 minutes.

For higher-intensity exercise of 45–50 minutes or more, or lower-intensity exercise lasting several hours, a sports drink can help maintain energy levels and its salt will improve hydration. Choose drinks that contain sodium (salt) when exercise lasts longer than one hour, or in any event when large amounts of salt will be lost through your sweat.

How do I stay motivated?

Make sure your exercise regime includes activities that you like doing rather than what someone else tells you to do. Exercise with a friend or friends so that you can all keep each other motivated.

'Set new challenges to keep yourself stimulated,' says Robin. 'And keep going. It's always hard at first, even for elite athletes, but it does get easier.'

16 July 2011

⇨ The above information is reprinted with kind permission from NHS Choices. Please visit www.nhs.uk for further information.

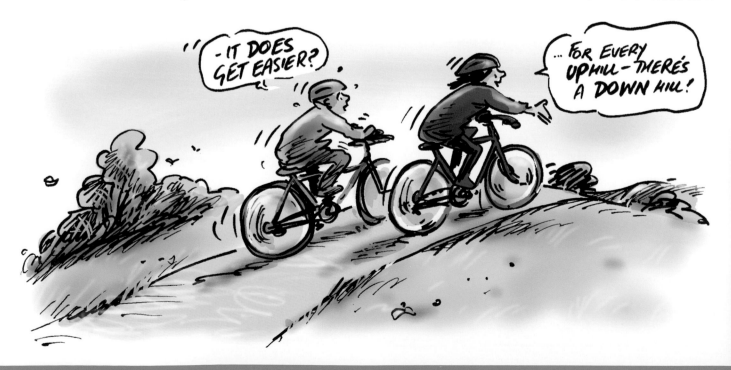

WORKOUT

Do quick workouts beat long ones?

Information from NHS Choices.

The secret of keeping fit is to 'do less exercise', says the *Daily Express*. The newspaper claims that new research shows that short bursts of intense activity are enough to keep most people fit, 'blowing away the myth that staying in shape takes hours of dedication'.

The news is based on a small study in seven healthy men, comparing their fitness levels before and after a two-week programme of short cycling sessions. After the course of six sessions the researchers found the men had improved exercise performance and metabolism in their muscles.

However, this study did not compare this exercise regime with others, or look at any long-term benefits of exercise, such as any reduction in heart disease or obesity. This, and other limitations, means the research does not support the claims that short bursts of intensive exercise offer as much benefit as the officially recommended, more frequent, but less intensive exercise. Government guidelines suggest 30 minutes of moderate-intensity exercise taken five times a week.

Where did the story come from?

This study was carried out by Dr Jonathan Little and colleagues from McMaster University in Canada. The research was funded by the Natural Sciences and Engineering Research Council of Canada and individual researchers were supported by grants from various health research organisations. The study was published in the peer-reviewed *Journal of Physiology*.

Newspapers have reported on the study in some detail, but most fail to discuss the shortcomings of this small, non-comparative study. A few do report that the short-term changes assessed in this study, muscle metabolic capacity and functional performance, do not equate with long-term cardiovascular health. This is very preliminary evidence towards the reported theory that 'less really can be more when it comes to exercise'.

What kind of research was this?

In this before-and-after experiment, seven men undertook six training sessions over a period of two weeks, with researchers comparing their performance and muscle health before the sessions with that seen after the training programme.

What did the research involve?

Seven healthy men were enrolled in this study. Their average age was 21, and they were reported to be healthy and 'recreationally active' two or three times a week, although none were 'engaged in a structured exercise training programme'. They were asked to maintain normal diet and routine levels of physical activity throughout the study but to refrain from any sporting activities beyond the exercise programme.

During each of their six exercise sessions (on Monday, Wednesday and Friday for two weeks), they did short bursts of high-intensity cycling. In each session they performed eight to 12 repetitions of a one-minute burst at 100% of their individual maximum power output (as determined by previous tests), followed by a recovery period, which was 75 seconds of low-intensity cycling. The time commitment for each training session was around 30 minutes including warm-up and recovery.

Timed cycling trials were used to assess the participants' exercise capacity 72 hours after the end of their final training session. Tissue samples were also taken from their 'skeletal muscle', the type of muscle tissue that powers movement and activities like running, walking and lifting. These tissue samples (taken from a muscle in the quadriceps) were assessed for their protein content and general metabolism and compared with a tissue sample taken prior to training.

'Current recommendations of 30 minutes' physical activity a day, five days a week, are based on rigorous reviewing of the evidence and discussion with experts.'

Researchers used a statistical test called a 'paired Student's t-test' to compare the participants' results after their training with their results prior to it. This is an appropriate statistical analysis method that takes into account the fact that this is a before-and-after study.

'Researchers found that the time taken to complete the cycling trials improved by about 10% after training.'

What were the basic results?

The researchers found that the time taken to complete the cycling trials improved by about 10% after training and that there was an increase in the average power during the trial. The activity of various enzymes in muscle cells also improved, as did the cells' protein content.

How did the researchers interpret the results?

The researchers say that the results of their study demonstrate that low volume HIT (high-intensity training) is a 'potent stimulus for increasing skeletal muscle [energy releasing] capacity and improving exercise performance'. They also say that the results shed light on ways in which exercise training potentially promotes changes in the metabolism in skeletal muscle.

Conclusion

This small observational study has demonstrated an improvement in muscle health following low-volume, high-intensity training in seven healthy men. There are a number of points to keep in mind when considering the results of this research, including:

⇨ The small sample size. The study included only seven men with an average age of 21. The researchers report that they were healthy and 'recreationally active two or three times a week', but that 'none were engaged in a structured exercise training programme'. The results of the study cannot therefore be taken to represent the wider population, particularly older people.

⇨ This study lacked a comparator group. While newspapers have reported that short bursts of high-intensity exercise are as effective as longer-term training is, the research featured no direct comparison between the two. Although the researchers say that their programme was 'designed to be more practical and attainable for the general population', they do not claim that their exercise programme was better than other types or durations of exercise.

⇨ Given that the participants were all healthy, active young men, it is likely that they were doing other forms of activity and exercise outside of their experimental training programme. The Department of Health recommendations on physical activity say that activities of daily life, including walking, gardening and cleaning, can all count as forms of exercise.

⇨ The Department of Health document *At least five a week* acknowledges that there is 'growing support for the benefits of accumulating activity in shorter bouts of activity of ten minutes or more, interspersed throughout the day', and reports that equivalent total volumes of short activities have demonstrated positive effects similar to a single, long bout of activity. This particular study, although using a weak

design, adds further evidence that low-volume, high-intensity training is good for muscles and their metabolism. However, how well it compares to other regimens is yet to be established.

⇨ Research needs to establish how suitable short bursts of intensive exercise are for different groups of people, particularly older people or people with health problems like arthritis or high blood pressure.

These findings are interesting, but it remains to be seen whether the improvements in muscle metabolism and exercise performance observed in this study are the same as those seen with other levels of exercise. Furthermore, it remains to be seen whether they will translate into the longer-term health benefits (such as reductions in heart disease, strokes and obesity) that are associated with the levels of exercise recommended by the Department of Health.

'it remains to be seen whether the improvements in muscle metabolism and exercise performance here are the same as those seen with other levels of exercise.'

While this type of research may suggest theoretical benefits to short bursts of intensive exercise, it does not change the fact that regular, moderate-intensity exercise is good for our health. The current recommendations of 30 minutes' physical activity a day, five days a week, are based on rigorous reviewing of the evidence and discussion with experts.

15 March 2010

⇨ Information from from NHS Choices. Please visit www.nhs.uk for further information.

Sporting poverty gap must be filled says McAllister

It is a sad fact of sporting life that areas with a below average household income have below average levels of participation and sports club membership.

Activity in rates in sport can see those in the highest social grade in Wales almost five times more likely to be a member of a sports club than those individuals sitting in the lowest grade.

But while that correlation might not be limited to sport, it is a trend that Wales' top sports administrator is keen to tackle.

'Whilst our Vision focuses on the improvement and development of Welsh sport it specifically recognises sports ability to positively influence an array of personal, community and nationwide developments,' commented Professor Laura McAllister, Chair of Sport Wales.

'Those of us who work in sport see these positive influences on a daily basis and can identify people and communities that sport has helped to unite and prosper.

'We are determined that the sporting sector will do everything it can to ensure opportunities are there for everyone, regardless of where they live.

'I have the same determination when it comes to getting more females and those from BME groups into volunteering or coaching. We must do our bit to ensure that it is as easy as possible to hook them into sport.'

And there are signs that new schemes are showing how they can make a dent in the sporting poverty gap.

In North Wales a cash injection from Sport Wales is helping families to get fit through sport in Wrexham's Caia Park Communities First area.

Organisers of the Caia Park Family Support Group were able to invest nearly £600 worth of Community Chest funding to buy badminton and rounders equipment and pay for an instructor to give weekly salsa taster sessions.

The sports and fitness sessions are aimed at boosting the confidence of families, and particularly mothers, from the estate who wouldn't normally take part in sport.

Pat Kearsley, from the Caia Park Family Support Group, said: 'We had a starter grant from Sport Wales earlier in the year to start fitness sessions and our members have absolutely loved it. It's taken off like a rocket!

'We've had a lot of help from the Caia Park Health Group, who have set up classes and lent us equipment. But

	A	B	C1	C2	D	E
Any participation	78%	72%	64%	57%	53%	35%
Any sports club membership	31%	28%	21%	16%	11%	6%
Any sports volunteering	15%	9%	6%	4%	3%	3%

Source: Active Adults Survey 2008/09

Social Grade	Chief income earner's occupation
A	Higher managerial, administrative or professional
B	Intermediate managerial, administrative or professional
C1	Supervisory or clerical and junior managerial, administrative or professional
C2	Skilled manual workers
D	Semi and unskilled manual workers
E	Casual or lowest grade workers, pensioners and others who depend on the welfare state for their income

members decided that if they had their own equipment then they could take part in sport whenever they wanted.

'This is part of a wider package, that includes cooking and nutrition classes, to help improve health in the Caia Park community. We also do a weigh in each week to give an added incentive and an element of competition.

'We've had parents bringing their older children along, which we hadn't anticipated, and we've even had a few dads along. So what started off as a small private exercise class has grown and we want to keep that momentum going.'

High levels of unemployment and long-term illness, combined with low income levels have plagued Blaenau Gwent in recent years, often putting sport at the bottom of the 'to do' list. But the introduction of StreetGames has utilised sport in tackling some of those wider community issues.

Running for just over two years, Blaenau Gwent County Borough Council introduced the programme to complement the already existing opportunities for young people to get involved in sport, but also to reach some of the disengaged youngsters within the community.

Whether down to lack of access to sporting opportunities, a lack of interest in traditional or mainstream sport or because they're from an area of high deprivation, StreetGames gets to the heart of the community and offers sport and physical activity to those youngsters not already involved in structured club sport, at the right time and price and in the right style.

And it certainly seems to be making its mark. To date, almost 2,500 individuals have participated in the sessions that take place at least once a week across 12 different sites across the borough.

From dance to basketball and predominantly multi-sport sessions, the activity most often takes place in the early evening during the week and also involves tournaments and festivals for those interested in the more competitive side of sport.

Gareth Gunter, Active Communities Officer at Blaenau Gwent County Borough Council, said;

'StreetGames was added to the sporting programme in Blaenau Gwent to help plug some of the gaps in participation in those areas of deprivation. Not only are we seeing encouraging numbers of youngsters taking part in the activities, we've also been able to enrich the lives of local young people through volunteering and coaching opportunities.

'52 volunteers have been involved in the programme so far, with 30 of those regularly running and contributing to sessions in their communities. We've been able to establish alternative volunteer programmes off the back of StreetGames, which in turn is helping to ensure that we can continue to provide sustainable opportunities.'

In south-west Wales, with boxing proving a popular choice of sport with youngsters, a former Commonwealth medallist is hoping his effort to get more women and girls involved will prove a knock-out.

The Prizefighter Gym in Carmarthen, owned by three-time Commonwealth Games medallist Kevin Evans, has been given a Sport Wales grant of £3,450 to get more young people, particularly women and girls, through the gym doors.

The National Lottery development grant funding will help purchase a new custom made-boxing ring, underlay and canvas, gloves, headguards, bags and pads.

It means the club can run new sessions for junior males and females and meet the growing demand.

The gym was opened by renowned boxer Evans in 2007 and has attracted members from Aberystwyth and Swansea, as well as from across Carmarthenshire.

'This is another step for us in improving what we offer at the gym,' said Evans.

'It means more equipment for those who want to come in and train and we can accommodate more people at the same time.

'We've made a commitment to try and get more youngsters through the door, which is one of the hopes I had when I first opened the gym. If I can get more youngsters interested in boxing, and produce some good fighters along the way, it goes a long way towards what I wanted to achieve.'

30 January 2012

⇨ The above information is reprinted with kind permission from Sport Wales. Please visit www.sportwales.org.uk for further information.

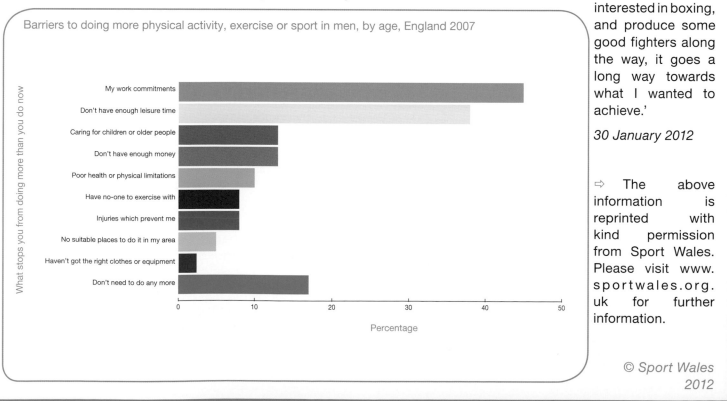

Barriers to doing more physical activity, exercise or sport in men, by age, England 2007

What stops you from doing more than you do now:
- My work commitments
- Don't have enough leisure time
- Caring for children or older people
- Don't have enough money
- Poor health or physical limitations
- Have no-one to exercise with
- Injuries which prevent me
- No suitable places to do it in my area
- Haven't got the right clothes or equipment
- Don't need to do any more

Percentage (0, 10, 20, 30, 40, 50)

'How I caught the running bug'

Aimee Albert talks about starting running, running to music and sharing her running goals on Facebook.

When did you first start running?

I started running about a month ago. I've never been any good at sport. As a child, I had mobility problems because of weak ankles and knees and that really held me back. I'd always thought 'I can't do sport'. But I just knew I had to start leading a healthier life while I was still young. I started doing exercises to strengthen my legs and then felt I could take it a bit further. I considered joining a gym but that's expensive so I decided to give running a go. Anyone can run. All you need is a pair of running shoes.

How did you get started?

I did a bit of research on running shoes. I spoke to friends who were runners and looked at websites like Runner's World. I was advised to go to a specialist running shop, where staff are trained to analyse your running style and help you choose the right pair of shoes. My local store had a treadmill, where they filmed me running to look at how my foot strikes the ground. They recommended some shoes – they're really comfy.

The next step was to search for music. I knew I didn't want to run with other people. I just wanted to get on with it by myself. I liked the idea of running to music and I was told you could get music specifically for running. I found the AudioFuel tracks on iTunes and bought Easy Beats, which is a gentle 30-minute walk and jog session with voiceover coaching.

Before setting off, I worked out my route using the Mapmyrun website so that I'd be home by the end of my session.

Describe your progress since starting running

Over the last month it's been great to find it less and less of a struggle to complete my 30-minute walking and jogging session. I've enjoyed it a lot more than I expected right from the start. I had a few aches in my legs after my runs in the beginning. That's normal but it doesn't last. I've definitely caught the running bug. Now I'm looking forward to making more progress. I want to run for longer although not necessarily faster.

How has the running music helped?

AudioFuel produce music to match your foot stride to the beat as you run. Running to the beat makes it easy to keep to the right pace and not tire myself out too quickly by setting off too fast. It's a nice feeling to be able to complete a 30-minute run. I didn't think I'd like the coaching. I thought it would be intrusive but it really works. I like the encouraging words and the timekeeping. It doesn't feel intrusive at all. It just keeps you motivated and focused.

How do you feel since starting running?

I don't get tired so much anymore. I now manage to run for the full half hour. I used to reach certain points on my run where I'd feel exhausted and want to stop but now I just keep going. I don't feel like stopping. I can see my progress.

I feel much better about myself now. I've taken action to improve my fitness. I've overcome my struggle with doing sport. Having always said to myself 'I can't', I'm now actually doing it, and I'm not bad at it which has been a real feelgood factor for me. I'm feeling fitter and more energetic.

Running's also really good for stress. When you go out for a run it all drops away and you stop feeling cross or worried. I don't care what I look like. I've lost my self-consciousness. Everyone looks hot and sweaty so it doesn't matter.

How do you fit running into your routine?

I like running in the evening. I'm not really a morning person. I tend to come home from work, put my shoes on and get out there. That's at around 6.30pm. It relaxes me after work and then I can have a nice relaxing bath afterwards.

Have you set yourself any goals?

I've signed up to do a 5km charity run with my sister-in-law. It's a Race for Life event to raise money for Cancer Research UK. I've got people sponsoring me. It's great to have a goal. It keeps me on track with my running every week because I can't let people down. But it's not high pressure – there's people of every fitness level who enter. On the day, I can walk, jog or run.

Any tips for new runners?

Get a good pair of shoes so you avoid injury. Then just get on and do it. It was raining on the day of my first run, and I just got on with it. Plan your runs at the start of each week and try to stick to a routine. Tell people you're going for a run today – your partner or your Facebook friends – then you can't get out of it. There are days when you'd rather collapse on the sofa with a cup of tea. Try to blank out those thoughts. Just put on some feelgood music while you get ready. Don't think about it too much and get on with it.

31 May 2012

⇨ The above information is reprinted with kind permission from NHS Choices. Please visit www.nhs.uk for further information.

Top tips to get you running for health

Running is a relatively simple way to get fit and is about as accessible as it gets. Just head out the door, and the streets themselves are your gym. You can even largely ignore the British summer.

And it has some great benefits. While it boosts the production of collagen in skin cells – keeping it firmer as you get older – jogging also builds bone strength, something that can really help keep your standard of life high as you age, warding off conditions such as osteoporosis according to *The Huffington Post*. And whatever your age, you could likely benefit from taking a more active life.

Thinking more long term, Level Term life insurance can provide a lump sum to help protect your family financially when you're gone, pay for your funeral expenses and help pay off any debts you might have – depending on your circumstances and the type of policy you choose.

But while running really can be as simple as putting on an old tracksuit and slipping into a decent pair of trainers, there are still some things to bear in mind. So if you were fired up by the spring marathon season, how do you best prime yourself for pavement-pounding this summer?

Easy does it

Before hitting the streets in earnest, assess where you are in terms of your fitness. If you are emerging from a period of inactivity, or perhaps recovering from winter flu or other illness, then you'll need to start off fairly easily. Consult your doctor if you have any health concerns before starting a new exercise regime.

A good way to progress is to mostly walk around a route to begin with, then to gradually increase the proportion you jog, until a couple of months in, when you can jog for around 15 minutes at a stretch.

In terms of frequency, three runs a week is a sustainable level, giving yourself a day to rest in between each session. Make sure you take care of yourself – and maximise the benefit of your workout – by warming up and down to reduce the risk of muscle strain or stiffness.

Just put one foot in front of the other?

Running is simple, right? Well, as with any sport, there is a technical element – albeit a fairly minor one. You'll need to think about your stride; try not to overstretch, for example, as this will mean you land heavily on your heel, and will actually slow you up. If you are prone to doing this, try upping your cadence to three steps per second.

Above all, try to remain relaxed when you run. Try leaning forward slightly from the waist – but still 'stand tall' without hunching your shoulders. Keep your head up, and avoid clenching your fists.

Health benefits

You may be lucky and really enjoy your running once you get into it, or you may simply view it as a means to an end. Whichever it is, you can be sure that there are a number of health benefits to jogging which run beyond the simple feeling of well-being which you will doubtless experience when you finish a session.

One of the first things you may notice is that, if you are unused to regular exercise, you may well feel less restless and therefore find it easier to sleep – though obviously try to avoid exercising too close to your normal bedtime, otherwise it may have the opposite effect, leaving you feeling wired when you should be winding down.

And while you should be better able to switch off at night, you should also experience an improvement in your ability to concentrate during the day, due to better oxygen and blood flow to the brain, along with an improved ability to cope with stress, and a natural boost in happiness – running stimulates the release of endorphins.

Of course, it's not just these 'mental' factors. One of the main benefits of jogging is the boost to your cardiovascular system. Getting the blood pumping as you run means a lowered risk of heart disease, diabetes and high blood pressure – just get out and work up a sweat.

Issued by Sainsbury's Bank

All information is correct at time of print. This may be subject to change. The views expressed in this editorial are those of the writer/blogger/journalist and not of Sainsbury's Bank plc or the Sainsbury's Group of Companies.

⇨ The above information is reprinted with kind permission from fitmap.co.uk. Please visit www.thefitmap.co.uk for further information.

© 2000-2008 thefitmap.co.uk

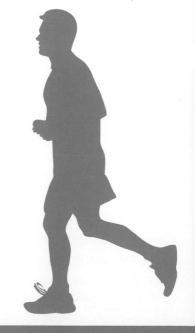

Keep dancing...

The health and well-being benefits of dance for older people.

Introduction

The older population in many parts of the world is growing rapidly and, at the same time, it is becoming more diverse. Recent projections suggest that, in England and Wales alone, by 2026 there will be over ten million people aged 65 and over, of whom 1.3 million will be from black and minority ethnic groups. As people age they tend to adopt an increasingly sedentary lifestyle but there is widespread and compelling evidence that increased levels of physical activity will improve both the longevity and the health of older people.[1] This report reviews the international evidence for the health benefits of dancing for older people.

Exercise programmes for older people commonly experience high drop-out rates. Dance, on the other hand, is an enjoyable and sociable form of exercise where participants report very high levels of motivation.[2]

Dance is also increasingly catching the public imagination. In 2010 over ten million viewers tuned in to watch episodes of the BBC1 TV programme *Strictly Come Dancing*. This increased interest in dance provides an opportunity to offer dance sessions for older people in community centres, care homes, village halls and hospitals across the country.

Local dance projects for older people have been set up in many parts of the UK. Similar programmes of dance, including ethnic dance, for older people, have been adopted worldwide including recreational dance in Australia.[3]

There are a number of benefits to dance for older people:

⇨ dance is inclusive and one of the principles of community dance for older people is that anyone and everyone can take part;[4]

⇨ dance can be tailored to match the physical capabilities of an older person and dance can also reflect the cultural diversity of the older population; and

⇨ dance is a social activity and, as such, can benefit both the physical health of older people and promote a sense of well-being and social inclusion.

Executive summary and key findings

This report identifies a number of issues around exercise for older people and draws together the key health benefits of dance for older people. These benefits can promote both physical and emotional well-being.

Older people don't get enough exercise

⇨ Only 20% of men and 17% women aged 65-74 get the recommended levels of physical exercise.

⇨ For people aged over 75 this falls to 9% for men and 6% for women.

This lack of exercise matters because taking part in physical activity improves both health and life expectancy

⇨ Regular physical activity by older people reduces the occurrence of a number of chronic conditions including cardiovascular disease, diabetes, cancer, hypertension, obesity, depression and osteoporosis.

⇨ Older people who engage in physical activity live longer and those who carry out more intense physical activity for longer periods live longest on average.

Dance benefits the body and the mind

⇨ Dance is a good source of aerobic exercise and a well-designed dance session can also provide low-level resistance exercise.

⇨ Dance has physical health benefits including improvements in balance, strength and gait, which help reduce the risk of falls, a significant health hazard in later life.

⇨ Dance has been shown to be beneficial in the direct treatment of a number of conditions including arthritis, Parkinson's disease, dementia and depression. Taking part in ballroom dancing has been shown to reduce the chances of getting dementia by 76%.

⇨ Taking part in dance also improves the mental health of older people including reaction times and cognitive performance.

Dance promotes emotional well-being of older people and combats isolation

⇨ Older people enjoy dance sessions and are more likely to continue to attend them – thereby gaining proportionately more physical benefits than they would from ordinary exercise sessions.

⇨ The social aspects of dance help to overcome feelings of social isolation and depression.

⇨ Dance is inclusive – there are no targets, and no failures, which contrasts with the philosophy of sports-based activities.

This report shows that there is considerable and emerging evidence of the benefits of dance as an exercise option for older people. However, too often policy makers in the Government and beyond are overlooking the contribution dance can make to the welfare of older people, often concentrating on less inclusive exercise and sports-based activities.

Bupa calls on policy makers to pay more attention to dance.

We believe that supporting organisations that provide dance activities for older people in the community, in care homes and hospitals, can make a major contribution to better physical and mental well-being of the growing numbers of older people in the population.

Dance as exercise

Dancing can take many forms. Most forms of dance will provide the opportunity for aerobic exercise – exercise that requires more than the usual day-to-day levels of exertion and causes increased heart and breathing rates, thus enhancing the body's ability to take in, transport and use oxygen.

Contemporary dance and some other forms of dance may, as well, allow the opportunity for some low-level resistance exercise – exercise that causes individual muscles to work against some form of resistance thereby increasing muscular strength. According to researchers 'it has been observed that dance-based aerobic exercise can improve the balance capacity, as well as the walking and agility profile of the older participant'.[5]

Some of the more energetic forms of dance, Cajun jitterbug, Irish set dance and Scottish country dancing for example, provide excellent aerobic exercise. Ballroom and Latin American dancing require good coordination and fluidity.[6]

With dance, the exercise gained, while important, is secondary to the dance experience as a whole. Nonetheless, the physical demands of the dance experience should be appropriate to the capabilities of the older person.

The Better Ageing Research Collaborative guidelines for exercise programming for older people suggest multiple components including warm-up, aerobic exercise, specific concentric and eccentric strengthening exercises, and exercises to improve co-ordination balance and flexibility/mobility (Tai Chi or similar). The guidelines recommend that aerobic exercise should be conducted at 60-80% maximum heart rate and resistance exercise should be targeted at eight to ten repetitions

on the large muscle groups, building from two to three sets over a period of 12 weeks.[7]

Recent reviews have drawn together evidence of the health advantages of dance for older people. These reviews offer compelling evidence that dance programmes for older people can have significant health benefits.[8]

One review considered the quality of the evidence and focused on studies that provide very strong or fairly strong evidence of the benefits or otherwise of dance as exercise for older people.[9] The review concluded that there is fairly strong scientific evidence that a dance-based exercise programme can improve older people's:

⇨ aerobic power;

⇨ muscle endurance of the lower extremities;

⇨ muscle strength of the lower extremities;

⇨ flexibility of the lower extremities;

⇨ static balance;

⇨ dynamic balance and agility; and

⇨ gait speed.

There is less strong evidence that dance-based exercise programmes for older people can also:

⇨ increase bone-mineral content in the lower body;

⇨ increase muscle power of the lower extremities;

⇨ reduce the rate of falls; and

⇨ reduce cardiovascular health risk.[10]

Dance is more than just exercise

Dance for older people provides more than just an opportunity for greater levels of aerobic or resistance exercise than might normally be experienced, and the associated health benefits that such exercise will bring.

Dance, perhaps especially dance with a partner, including ballroom dancing and many forms of traditional folk dance, is a social experience with the mental-health benefits that can come from social involvement and avoiding social isolation.

Many forms of dancing, including ballroom dancing, require high levels of concentration and co-ordination

with the mental-health advantages that can follow from increased levels of focused mental activity over a sustained period.

Dance is an enjoyable experience so that, in addition to the general improvement in an individual's sense of well-being that dance activity brings, dance programmes experience relatively low drop-out rates. As a result, older people gain proportionately greater exercise and other benefits overall from a dance programme.

Some forms of dance provide the opportunity for self-expression and the mental health benefits that can follow from a sense of mental liberation and the release of tension.

Traditional folk dance, including Scottish and Irish country dance and traditional Greek or Turkish dance, may reawaken a sense of the cultural identity of youth for some older people with benefits similar to reminiscence and memory therapy.

Older people taking part in dance groups that have a performance outcome find additional satisfaction in a successful performance and the sense of purpose that the end performance provides to the dance experience.

References

1 Lievesley, 2010; Health Survey for England, 2008

2 Nordin and Hardy, 2009

3 Connor, 2000

4 Houston, 2005

5 Marks, 2005 referencing Judge, 2003

6 Bremer, 2007

7 Better Ageing Research Collaborative, 2005

8 Keogh et al (2009), Trinity Laban Conservatoire of Music and Dance (2011) and Dance South West and the Department of Health (2011)

9 Keogh et al, 2009a

10 Keogh et al. 2009b

⇨ The above information is reprinted with kind permission from Bupa. Please visit www.bupa.co.uk for further information.

As obesity levels rise, scheme has one goal to get kids off the sofa and fighting fit

In 40 years, 90 per cent of the population of the UK will be overweight or obese.

It is a shocking statistic and a growing trend that appears nigh on unstoppable.

The big problem is inactivity among children.

The children of the PlayStation generation do far less exercise than their parents or grandparents, and it is beginning to show.

In the 1970s, children grew up in an active and mainly healthy environment. They walked to school, and played in the playground.

Fast forward 40 years and fast food outlets and computer gaming have become key pastimes for children.

And physical fitness of children is declining by nine per cent a decade.

The latest data shows that obesity in North Lincolnshire is above the national average.

Statistics released earlier this year showed an estimated 27,000 adults in the region (26.9 per cent) to be obese. This was the highest level in the Yorkshire and Humber region.

Figures from NHS North Lincolnshire do show more than seven per cent of children aged five to six are still at risk of obesity, with another 11.6 per cent assessed as at risk of being overweight.

The picture for older children shows over 66 per cent assessed as being of a healthy weight. This is the same as the national average for children aged ten to 11, but it does mean almost one in five children of this age are assessed as being at risk of obesity. An additional 13.2 per cent of 11-year-olds in North Lincolnshire were assessed as overweight.

Now staff at Project HE:RO (Health Engagement:Real Outcomes) aim to change that.

The scheme, run by the not-for-profit organisation Evolve Sport, inspires primary schoolchildren to be more active and tries to get them involved in sport.

It has proved popular at schools in Scunthorpe, as have events like Saturday Soccer, held every week at Premier Pitches on Kettering Road.

'But that's only about three per cent of what we do,' said Graham Morgan, director at Evolve.

'What we're trying to do is prevent obesity levels from rising. But we're getting far more exciting results than we anticipated.

'The teachers are telling us that attendance and attainment levels are rising.

'The question is "what are we doing to our children?" They didn't ask to be born, we bring them into the world, and we put them in a system that's based on academic attainment and not health.

'We need to educate for a healthier future and that's exercise, cooking healthier meals, cutting down on smoking and alcohol consumption.

'There are all these things that can damage a life, and we're trying to inspire children to realise that their lives are very important.

'The current kids in school, by 2050, 90 per cent of them will be overweight or obese. That 90 per cent will be more than enough to bankrupt the NHS.

'But if you're teaching a six-year-old in school today then that's really hard to worry about because they're going to leave and they're not going to become overweight on your watch.'

It is a challenge that Damon Fox, regional manager for Evolve Sport in Lincolnshire, is experiencing first-hand.

'The problem is that now when I'm talking to headteachers about inactivity and obesity, they look out to their classrooms and they don't see a lot of fat children.

'It's not a problem for them at the moment, but we're trying to prevent what's going to happen in ten years.

'Our focus is getting more people active and that has to start with the kids, because by the age of ten they've decided what their traits will be like, whether they will play football or do dance, or smoke or whatever.'

Damon says Evolve has worked in at least 60 per cent of schools in Scunthorpe, as well as running Saturday Soccer.

'Our focus is in school time,' he said. 'We've got health mentors who are young, fit and sporty and the kids want to be like them.

'The feedback from teachers is very positive and the parents are very keen on it too.

'Inactivity is our focus, not obesity as such. At breaks and dinner-times, a lot of children just sit around and don't do anything.'

Health mentors try to stimulate kids and get them excited about doing exercise and socialising with each other, be that in the playground or during a PE lesson.

Outside of school, dozens of kids turn up for Saturday Soccer.

It has impressed many. Mark Goulding brought his three boys Kieran, ten, Declan, seven, and Corey, four, along to Premier Pitches last weekend.

'It's the first time I've brought my youngest but I think it's absolutely sound,' he said.

'It's great for the kids. They'd be sat at home or playing in the streets, kicking a football on the road otherwise and that's not really safe.'

Playing football in the street is at least still active, although Kieran said he probably would have been sitting at home.

'It's pretty good here,' he said.

'I'd probably be bored at home if I wasn't here, or in my room playing Xbox.'

Lee Woffinden saw his son Dylan, six, pick up a star player award – a helpful incentive that Damon started.

'We've just signed up for another ten weeks and he loves it,' said Lee.

'He comes off sweating and having enjoyed himself, especially today after he got star player.'

Dylan said the award made him want to come back each week.

'I like getting star player and, if I try my best, then maybe I'll get it again next week,' he said.

'I get to play with my friends and run about and make some new friends, and I'm learning how to play football.'

However, there is more to staying fit and healthy than just exercise.

Earlier this week, a leading surgeon told the Government they should stop promoting exercise as a key way to tackle the obesity epidemic.

Tory Lord McColl of Dulwich, professor and director of surgery at Guy's Hospital in London for 27 years until his retirement in 1998, said eating less rather than greater activity was the crucial factor in losing weight.

'We are in the middle of the most serious epidemic to have hit this country for 100 years – the obesity epidemic,' he said at question time in the House of Lords.

'The cure is free – you just have to eat less.'

19 September 2011

⇨ The above information is reprinted with kind permission from the *Scunthorpe Telegraph*. Please visit www.thisisscunthorpe.co.uk for further information.

Outdoor fitness equipment: taking the 'play' out of the playground?

Recently there seems to have been an increase in the number of parks that have outdoor 'gyms', with more and more community parks sprouting pieces of specialised equipment designed to encourage adults to be active.

By Sally Pears

In theory, these 'adult playgrounds' sound like a great idea:

⇨ They're free: for anyone put off by the cost of gym memberships or home equipment, free outdoor gyms are a great alternative.

⇨ They're outside: perfect for anyone who doesn't have space at home to workout, or who wants to get out in the fresh air and maybe get some sun (not that we've had much of that here in the UK lately).

⇨ They're a good exercise reminder: acting as a prompt to anyone walking past that they should maybe get a little more exercise.

⇨ They're inexpensive: As far as public health interventions, outdoor gyms are relatively cheap – there's a one-off payment for the equipment and that's it – no fees for staff, no printing/advertising costs, etc.

BUT, how effective are these outdoor gyms in practice, really? Personally, I think there are a number of reasons why investing public money in outdoor fitness equipment isn't the best idea:

1. No privacy

For anyone wanting to get fitter/get in shape, an outdoor gym probably comes a close second to donning a swimsuit in terms of potential for embarrassment. Many people often claim that they dislike gyms because they feel embarrassed about working out in public, so working out in a community park (surrounded by children, teenagers, dog walkers, etc.) would probably not be a good alternative!

2. No instruction

Again, for anyone starting out, these workout spaces provide very little instruction about how to use the equipment. Sure, each piece of kit may come with a sign explaining how to use it and what it's good for (e.g. cardiovascular conditioning, leg strength, balance, etc.) but there's rarely any information about how to put everything together – for example, how long should you do each exercise for, how many exercises should you do in one session, how often should you do the exercises. This might seem to take the 'fun' out of using the equipment, but another barrier to exercise often cited by people is that they don't know what to do! Providing free equipment is therefore only one half of the solution.

3. They just make no sense!

Okay, so this is my biggest argument against these outdoor 'gyms'. Most of the ones that I have seen have at least one or two pieces of equipment that are designed to mimic the 'cardio' machines found in fitness centres. Now, call me crazy, but surely you have to question the sense of producing specialised outdoor equipment that mimics gym equipment… which was itself originally designed to mimic the kind of activities that people do outdoors! For example:

⇨ An outdoor 'treadmill' (i.e. steel rollers that you 'run' on) mimics an indoor treadmill which mimics walking or running!

⇨ An outdoor stationary bike mimics an indoor stationary bike which mimics cycling!

⇨ An 'air walker' mimics the beloved cross-trainer which mimics… well, I never really have managed to figure out what movement a cross-trainer is designed to imitate!

I mean, come on! You're in a PARK! If you want to encourage people to exercise, what about providing them with actual bikes? Or setting up a walking or running group? Or even a setting up a frisbee golf course?!

Now, okay, some of you may agree that providing outdoor cardio equipment might not be the best idea, but surely there's a place for outdoor resistance machines like a shoulder press, chest press or leg press?

Well, I don't know if you've ever come across any outdoor resistance machines, but on the whole they actually offer very little actual 'resistance', mainly because it's tricky to provide an adjustable outdoor machine which won't

rust excessively or need regular maintenance, but also because it's generally considered unsafe to provide heavy weights to the (unsupervised) general public. So, given that the 'resistance' machines don't actually offer much resistance, why not just encourage people to use their own bodyweight instead:

⇨ Chest Press? – Why not a push up?

⇨ Shoulder Press? – Why not a pike push up?

⇨ Leg Press? – Why not a squat?

The same goes for machines like the 'twist plate' that are designed to improve hip mobility – what about good, old-fashioned hip circles? Or multi-planar lunges?

The solution?

I really do appreciate the councils are genuinely trying to encourage people to be more physically active and I definitely think that money invested in physical activity promotion/interventions could bring significant savings in terms of NHS costs. However, I think that money spent on outdoor cardio equipment and

resistance machines is just a waste of resources. But what's the alternative?

Personally, I would love to see some money spent on creating outdoor 'gyms' for adults which not only provide areas and advice on bodyweight exercises, but that also put the 'play' back into 'playgrounds' with balance beams, monkey bars, cargo nets and zip wires!

What are your thoughts on this issue and what physical activity promotion programmes do YOU think would be a good idea?

23 October 2012

⇨ The above information is reprinted with kind permission from *Fitness Newspaper.* Please visit www.fitnessnewspaper. com for further information.

© 2012 Fitness Newspaper

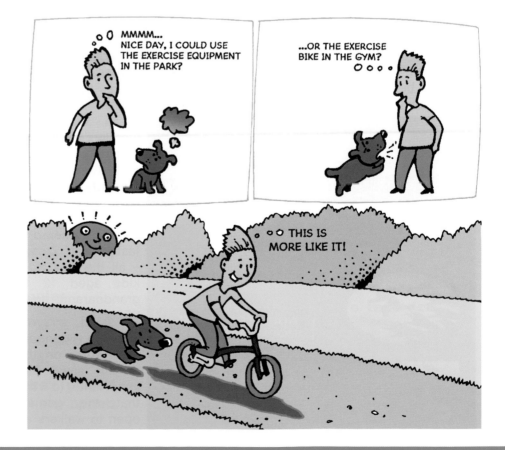

Key facts

⇨ Regular physical activity can reduce the risk of many chronic conditions including coronary heart disease, stroke, type 2 diabetes, cancer, obesity, mental health problems and musculoskeletal conditions. (page 1)

⇨ Everybody should aim to be active daily. For adults, the recommended amount is 150 minutes (2.5 hours) of moderate activity per week, in bouts of ten minutes or more. The overall amount of activity is more important than the type, intensity or frequency, and one way to achieve this is to do 30 minutes on at least five days a week. (page 1)

⇨ Physical activity levels are low in the UK: only 40% of men and 28% of women meet the minimum recommendations for physical activity in adults. (page 1)

⇨ Physically active people have a 20-30% reduced risk of premature death and up to 50% reduced risk of major chronic disease such as coronary heart disease, stroke and cancer. (page 2)

⇨ Obesity reduces life expectancy on average by nine years. (page 3)

⇨ Regular physical activity improves mood, helps relieve depression, and increases feelings of well-being. A survey carried out by the charity Mind found that 83% of people with mental health problems looked to physical activity to help lift their mood. (page 4)

⇨ Malta was the laziest country worldwide, with 72 per cent of adults classified as physically inactive, but Britain (63%) far outstretched other countries like the USA (41%), France (33%) and Greece (16%). (page 7)

⇨ Higher consumption of fruit and vegetables and lower consumption of crisps, sweets and fizzy drinks were both associated with high happiness. (page 8)

⇨ Mind's research found women were more likely to eat comfort food (71%), listen to sad music (32%), spend time social networking (57%), go to bed (66%) or find a way to be alone (71%), than exercise. (page 11)

⇨ According to Mind's survey, out of the women questioned, it was revealed that 60% are nervous about how their body reacts to exercise – their wobbly bits, sweating, passing wind or going red. (page 11)

⇨ New research by YouGov for Slimming World has found that nearly half of adults in the UK (45%) believe it would be difficult or impossible to run 100 metres without stopping. (page 13)

⇨ If two overweight or obese people have the same BMI, the person with a bigger waist circumference will be at a greater risk of developing health problems due to their weight. This is because it is not just whether you are carrying excess fat but where you are carrying it. The risks to your health are greater if you mainly carry a lot of extra fat around your waist ('apple-shaped'), rather than mainly on your hips and thighs ('pear-shaped'). (page 14)

⇨ Less than one in 100 obese people has a 'medical' cause for their obesity. For example, conditions such as Cushing's syndrome and an underactive thyroid are rare causes of weight gain. (page 16)

⇨ People with a BMI of 25 or more are considered overweight while those with a BMI of over 30 are obese. (page 17)

⇨ Almost a quarter of adults in England are obese (with a body mass index (BMI) of 30 or over). Around 800,000 are 'morbidly obese' – with a BMI of 40 or higher, the level at which life insurance companies may decline cover. (page 18)

⇨ An oft-quoted Foresight report predicted that the direct economic costs of overweight and obesity would be £6.4 billion a year by 2015. (page 18)

⇨ Nearly a third (31%) of children aged two to 15 are overweight or obese. (page 19)

⇨ It's important to drink fluid during any exercise that lasts for more than 30 minutes. (page 26)

⇨ Areas with a below average household income have below average levels of sport participation and sports club membership. (page 29)

BMI (body mass index)

An abbreviation which stands for 'body mass index' and is used to determine whether an individual's weight is in proportion to their height. If a person's BMI is below 18.5 they are usually seen as being underweight. If a person has a BMI greater than or equal to 25, they are classed as overweight and a BMI of 30 and over is obese. As BMI is the same for both sexes and adults of all ages, it provides the most useful population-level measure of overweight and obesity. However, it should be considered a rough guide because it may not correspond to the same degree of 'fatness' in different individuals (e.g. a body builder could have a BMI of 30 but would not be obese because his weight would be primarily muscle rather than fat).

Exercise intensity

This refers to how hard you exercise. Exercise intensity can be broken down into light, moderate or vigorous. Light exercise intensity feels easy; you have no noticeable changes in your breathing pattern and don't break a sweat. Moderate exercise intensity feels somewhat hard; your breath quickens and you develop a sweat after about ten minutes of activity (e.g. leisurely cycling, brisk walk, gardening) Vigorous exercise intensity feels very challenging; you can't carry on a conversation due to deep, rapid breathing and you develop a sweat after a few minutes of activity (e.g. jumping rope, basketball, running).

Fitness

The condition of being physically healthy (e.g. described as being in shape). Remember, fitness can also apply to our mental health and well-being. A high level of fitness is usually the result of regular exercise and a proper nutrition regime.

Obesity

When someone is obese, they have a BMI of 30 or over. This puts them at risk for a number of serious health problems, such as an increased risk of heart disease and type 2 diabetes. Worldwide obesity has more than doubled since 1980 and this is most likely due to our more sedentary lifestyle, combined with a lack of physical exercise.

Olympic legacy

This focuses on the idea that the London 2012 Olympics will help to inspire a new generation of aspiring athletes. It also refers to the new facilities that were built to cater for the Olympics, in the hope that they will be used after the Games and continue to grow businesses and help to regenerate the area. For example, the Olympic and Paralympic Village will be converted into thousands of new homes for people to buy and to rent. Visit www.london2012.com to find out more.

Physical activity

Physical activity includes all forms of activity, such as walking or cycling, active play, work-related activity, active recreation such as working out in a gym, dancing, gardening or competitive sport like football. Regular physical activity can reduce the risk of many chronic health conditions including coronary heart disease, type 2 diabetes, cancer and obesity. Regular physical activity also has positive benefits for mental health as it can reduce anxiety and enhance moods and self-esteem, which reduces the risk of depression.

Strength-training

Strength-training activities involve short bursts of effort which results in burning calories whilst building and strengthening muscle. This includes activities such as free weights, weight machines or activities that use your own body weight – such as rock climbing or heavy gardening. The benefits of strength training include increasing bone density, strengthening joints and improving balance, stability and posture. It is recommended that a person should do strength training exercises at least twice a week.

Weight loss surgery

Bariatric (weight-loss) surgery procedures are normally carried out on adults, but in some extreme cases this type of surgery may be considered for children. Weight loss surgery can provide a lasting solution for a wide range of obesity-related problems including diabetes, sleep apnoea and bone or liver disorders. The most common weight loss surgery is a gastric band operation. This is where an elastic band is fitted across the top end of the stomach to restrict the amount of food the person can eat before feeling full. Weight loss surgery is a major medical procedure and shouldn't be viewed as a quick fix; patients must maintain a strict diet and exercise regime after having the procedure (a person can typically expect to lose between 30 per cent and 50 per cent of their excess body weight). After-care is also important, with the patient having to undergo an intensive treatment programme with a dietician and a psychologist.

Assignments

1. Did you know that 'Half of people in UK cannot run 100 metres' (page 13)? Run 100 metres and time how long it takes you. What level of physical activity do you think you felt while running? Low, moderate or high?

2. 'The number of obese people in the UK is rising, particularly among young adults. Since 1980, the number of obese adults in the UK has nearly tripled. This has been called the obesity epidemic.' What is 'the obesity epidemic'? Why is this an important issue we must address in society today? Research different facts and statistics about obesity and present them in graphs, charts, drawings or any other way that you think will show the information best. Share with your class.

3. Research a new sport or fitness activity that you have always wanted to know more about. The more obscure the better! For example, have you ever considered archery or perhaps roller derby? Design a PowerPoint presentation that will persuade people to take-up this unique sport.

4. Has technology helped or hindered fitness? Take into account ideas such as the Wii Fit, fitness gadgets such as heart-rate monitors, and how children are spending more time watching TV rather than going outdoors. Write an article explaining your opinion.

5. Create a leaflet for your local health centre informing people of the recommended physical activity guidelines for each different age group: early years (under-fives), children and young people (five-18 years), adults (19-64 years) and older adults (65+ years). Offer examples for each age-group of activities they might try.

6. Recently there seems to have been an increase in the number of parks that have outdoor 'gyms', with more and more community parks sprouting pieces of specialised equipment designed to encourage adults to be active. Read 'Outdoor fitness equipment: Taking the "play" out of the playground?' on page 36. Do you think these outdoor fitness playgrounds are a good idea or bad idea? Would you use one? Discuss this with a partner.

7. What is the Olympic Games legacy? Do you think the London 2012 Olympics legacy will inspire and benefit a new generation of athletes? Read 'Fred Turok, chair of the Physical Activity Network talks about the Olympic legacy' on page 9 and 'London 2012 Olympic Games legacy "non-existent", says medalist Liz McColgan' on page 10. Consider the arguments that both articles present and write a summary, including your own opinion on the matter.

8. Read 'Keep dancing...' on page 33. Sum up this article and highlight the health and well-being benefits of dance for older people. Remember to consider dance as a social experience with mental health benefits too.

9. With a partner, debate the following motion: 'Sport in school should be compulsory.' One of you should argue in favour of the idea, the other against.

10. Find out about opportunities for young people to take part in sport outside of school in your local area. Write an article for your local magazine giving information on these opportunities and explaining how people can participate.

11. 'People spend too much time playing computer game versions of sports and not enough time out doing the real thing.' Do you think this is true? Write an essay analysing your views.

12. Nicole, a 14-year-old school girl, really enjoys playing basketball, but her friends have decided that they no longer want to play because they are embarrassed by the boys watching them, and becoming too sweaty. How can Nicole find a way to make PE less intimidating and encouraging to her female friends? Try and address the reasons why some girls are not that into PE lessons and how these issues can be solved so they can pursue fitness into later life. Discuss in groups.

13. Look at the graph on page 4 which demonstrates physical activity levels in different countries within the UK. Which country has the highest levels of physical activity? Why do you think this is? Why do you think people become less active as adults? Brainstorm your ideas and create a mind-map to demonstrate them.

14. The National Trust has launched a nationwide campaign to encourage sofa-bound children to get outside: 'National Trust: 50 things to do before you are 11 3/4.' Visit www.50things.org.uk and see how many activities on the list you have done. Which ones would you like to do next? Think of some more ideas that could be added to the list to encourage people, of all ages, to go outside and explore the outdoors more.

15. Read 'Zombie fitness app a runaway success for UK business' on page 38. Using this article for inspiration, create your own fitness app aimed towards the younger generation to help them get motivated and interested in exercise.

Acknowledgements

The publisher is grateful for permission to reproduce the following material.

While every care has been taken to trace and acknowledge copyright, the publisher tenders its apology for any accidental infringement or where copyright has proved untraceable. The publisher would be pleased to come to a suitable arrangement in any such case with the rightful owner.

Chapter One: Introduction to fitness

Physical activity and health © Sustrans 2012, Start active, stay active © Crown copyright 2011, British people among laziest in Europe © Telegraph Media Group Limited 2012, New research shows that healthy teenagers are happy teenagers © PSHE Association 2012, Fred Turok, chair of the physical activity network talks about the Olympic legacy © Crown copyright 2012, London 2012 Olympic Games legacy 'non-existent', says medalist Liz McColgan © The Independent, New findings show women run scared from outdoor exercise © 2012 Mind, Half of people in UK cannot run 100 metres © 2000-2012 YouGov plc.

Chapter Two: Obesity

Obesity in adults © EMIS 2011, Fat but fit: obese people can be healthy and in good metabolic shape © 2012 Christopher Hughes, The true financial cost of obesity © 2004-2012 SquareDigital Media Ltd, Childhood obesity © Royal College of Paediatrics and Child Health 2007-2012, New UK obesity centre offers surgery to teens © The Independent, Obese children to be put up for adoption © Telegraph Media Group Limited 2011, The NHS jobsworths employed to brand kids as fat © Adam Collyer 2011.

Chapter Three: Be active, get involved

Fitness training tips © NHS Choices 2011, Do quick workouts beat long ones? © NHS Choices 2010, Sporting poverty gap must be filled says McAllister © Sport Wales 2012, 'How I caught the running bug' © NHS Choices 2012, Top tips to get you running for health © 2000-2008 thefitmap.co.uk, Keep dancing... © Bupa 2011, As obesity levels rise, scheme has one goal to get kids off the sofa and fighting fit © 2011 Northcliffe Media Limited, Outdoor fitness equipment: taking the 'play' out of the playground? © 2012 Fitness Newspaper, Zombie fitness app a runaway success for UK business © Nesta 2012.

Illustrations:

Pages 3, 35: Don Hatcher; pages 9, 37: Angelo Madrid; pages 16, 38: Simon Kneebone.

Images:

Cover and pages i, 20, © Anthia Cumming, page 2 © Sanja Gienero, page 7 © Alex Raths, page 16 © Tony Alter, page 24 © Bowden Images, page 27 © G W Photographics, pages 38 and 39 © Zombies Run Game.

Additional acknowledgements:

Editorial on behalf of Independence Educational Publishers by Cara Acred.

With thanks to the Independence team: Mary Chapman, Sandra Dennis, Christina Hughes, Jackie Staines and Jan Sunderland.

Cara Acred

Cambridge, January 2013